THE
OUTLIVE DIET
NATURAL REMEDIES
ENCICLOPEDYA

Over 500 Herbal Healing Remedies and Natural Recipes Inspired
by Peter Attia's Teachings for a Long and Healthy Life

PATRICK NEEL

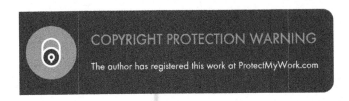

TABLE OF CONTENTS

Foreword

Welcome, my dear friend. As you begin this exploration of "The Outlive Natural Remedies Encyclopedia," you might wonder, "What makes this book different?" Allow me to share my journey—a narrative not of sudden transformations, but of a gradual, meaningful embrace of a life enriched by nature's potent gifts and the rigorous insights of longevity science.

For years, I navigated a landscape cluttered with conflicting health advice, where optimal wellness seemed elusive. Like many, I sought clarity and truth, a path that eventually led me to the principles of longevity and health optimization championed by those dedicated to understanding how we can live longer, healthier lives. This exploration was not about finding a quick fix but about embracing a lifestyle deeply rooted in the best practices of both traditional wisdom and scientific research.

This book is born out of the realization that natural remedies offer more than just health benefits—they are a way to profoundly connect with the body's natural healing processes. The philosophy you will discover here, inspired by the meticulous approach of Dr. Peter Attia, emphasizes the prevention of disease, the enhancement of metabolic health, and a deep dive into the science of aging. Dr. Attia's work has shown us that the key to longevity lies not only in treating symptoms but in fostering an environment within our bodies that promotes thriving health.

Here, you will find a curated collection of natural remedies that align with this holistic approach. These are not just recipes; they are gateways to better health and a more vibrant life. They support the body's inherent strengths and address its weaknesses with gentle, natural interventions that work in harmony with its complex systems.

Who am I to guide you on this journey? I am someone who has personally felt the transformative impact of integrating these natural remedies into my own life—guided by the rigorous, thoughtful approach to health maintenance that Dr. Attia advocates. I have experienced firsthand how powerful such changes can be and how accessible they are to everyone.

As we turn these pages together, I invite you to view them as a bridge between the world of natural healing and the cutting-edge science of living well. This book is more than a guide; it is a companion in your journey towards a longer, healthier life. Here, you will discover how to harness the benefits of the natural world in ways that science supports and respects.

So, with a heart open to new beginnings and a mind eager to explore the depths of natural healing, let's embark on this journey together. Let's learn, grow, and thrive as we unlock the secrets to a life well-lived, inspired by the enduring wisdom of nature and the transformative science of longevity.

INTRODUCTION

Overview of Peter Attia's Philosophy

Welcome to a world where longevity and optimal health are not just aspirations but achievable goals. This book is inspired by the philosophy of preventive medicine and health optimization, a philosophy that Peter Attia has articulated and practiced with profound commitment. Attia's approach is deeply analytical, combining the rigor of medical science with a passionate advocacy for proactive wellness. He teaches that to truly thrive, one must understand the complex interactions within our bodies and the impacts of our lifestyle choices.

Attia's methodology isn't about seeking immortality but about making your years as healthy and fulfilling as possible. He emphasizes the importance of metabolic health, mental resilience, and physical robustness, believing that the path to longevity is built on the foundation of these critical elements. His advocacy for a data-driven approach to diet, exercise, and sleep has revolutionized how we think about aging and disease prevention.

Increase Longevity

The pursuit of longevity is more than just delaying the inevitable; it's about enhancing the quality of life and ensuring that our later years are lived in good health. According to Attia, the key to increasing longevity lies in meticulously managing our metabolic processes, optimizing nutrition, and rigorously incorporating physical activity into our daily routines. He also highlights the critical role of managing stress and ensuring restorative sleep, all aimed at reducing the wear and tear of our biological systems over time.

This guide takes these core principles and translates them into practical, natural remedies and lifestyle adjustments that can be seamlessly integrated into your daily life. From nutritional advice that syncs with your body's needs to herbal supplements that support systemic health, each suggestion is backed by scientific insight and aimed at prolonging your healthspan.

How This Guide Will Meet Your Needs

Whether you are new to the concept of health optimization or someone who has been following Peter Attia's teachings for years, this guide is designed to meet you where you are. It offers a comprehensive look at natural remedies that can support and enhance Attia's health principles, providing you with practical tools to implement these strategies in your everyday life.

Each section of this book is crafted to help you understand how specific natural ingredients, herbs, and lifestyle practices can contribute to your longevity goals. It breaks down complex scientific concepts into actionable advice that can be applied to improve your metabolic health, enhance your physical stamina, and support your mental clarity.

By integrating the wisdom of traditional healing practices with the latest in scientific research, this guide empowers you to take charge of your health journey. It is a resource for those who seek to extend their healthspan and live a life characterized not just by years, but by vibrant, active, and purposeful living.

As you embark on this journey through the pages of this book, remember that each step you take brings you closer to a fuller, healthier life. Let this guide be your companion as you navigate the path of longevity, equipped with the knowledge and tools to thrive.

CHAPTER

01

UNDERSTANDING
NATURAL REMEDIES

Embracing Nature's Pharmacy

Natural remedies represent a profound connection between our health and the natural world. In this chapter, we explore how these ancient healing practices align with modern longevity philosophies, particularly focusing on the comprehensive, science-backed approach advocated by leaders in the field of health optimization like Peter Attia. Natural remedies involve using plants, herbs, minerals, and other naturally occurring substances to treat ailments, enhance well-being, and support bodily functions—ideals that perfectly complement a lifestyle aimed at achieving prolonged health and vitality.

The Science of Natural Remedies

While often passed down through generations as part of traditional medicine, many natural remedies have now been validated by scientific research for their efficacy and mechanisms of action. For instance, compounds like curcumin in turmeric and omega-3 fatty acids found in fish oil have been extensively studied for their anti-inflammatory and antioxidant properties. These natural compounds help mitigate the chronic inflammation and oxidative stress that Peter Attia identifies as key drivers of aging and metabolic diseases.

The longevity philosophy embraces the use of such substances not just for their symptom-alleviating effects but for their role in systemic health enhancement. This approach sees natural remedies as tools to optimize the body's functions—aiding everything from metabolic health to cognitive function, aligning closely with the goal of extending healthspan.

Integrating Natural Remedies into Modern Life

Incorporating natural remedies into our daily regimen involves more than just replacing pharmaceuticals with herbs or supplements. It requires a holistic understanding of how these substances interact with our bodies and how they can be synergistically combined with modern medical practices to promote longevity. For example, adopting a diet rich in natural, anti-inflammatory foods while also engaging in scientifically endorsed practices like intermittent fasting or targeted exercise can amplify the health benefits of each.

This synergy between traditional remedies and modern science offers a powerful strategy for those seeking to live longer, healthier lives. It allows individuals to proactively manage their health using a combination of the best that both worlds have to offer.

Practical Applications for Everyday Health

To truly harness the power of natural remedies in the pursuit of longevity, one must understand how to apply these principles practically:

- Dietary Adjustments: Incorporating foods rich in antioxidants, vitamins, and minerals that support cellular health and reduce inflammation.

- Herbal Supplementation: Using scientifically supported herbs and plants to enhance physiological functions, from boosting immune response to enhancing sleep quality.

◻ Lifestyle Modifications: Aligning sleep, stress management, and physical activity with natural circadian rhythms to maximize recovery and energy utilization.

Conclusion

Understanding and utilizing natural remedies is not just about treating ailments but about fostering an environment within our bodies that promotes optimal functioning and delays the onset of age-related decline. By aligning the wisdom of traditional medicine with the rigorous insights provided by longevity science, we equip ourselves with a potent set of tools designed to extend our healthful years and enhance our life quality.

In embracing these natural strategies, informed by the longevity principles of experts like Peter Attia, we not only seek to live longer but also ensure that our extended years are marked by vitality and robust health. This chapter sets the foundation for a deeper exploration of specific remedies and practices that you can incorporate into your life to achieve these goals.

02

HERBAL HEALING REMEDIES AND NATURAL RECIPES

Welcome to the heart of our exploration into the power of natural healing: Chapter 2 delves into a curated collection of herbal healing remedies and natural recipes designed to nourish, heal, and optimize your health in alignment with longevity principles. Here, we merge ancient herbal wisdom with the latest scientific research to create practical, everyday applications that support your quest for a longer, healthier life.

In this chapter, we not only provide recipes but also explain how these remedies can be seamlessly integrated into your daily routine to address specific health concerns, enhance bodily functions, and contribute to your overall well-being. Each remedy and recipe has been carefully selected for its potential to support the body's natural healing processes, boost immune function, improve metabolic health, and enhance mental clarity—all of which are foundational to achieving a prolonged healthspan.

As we proceed, you'll discover how simple it can be to harness the therapeutic powers of herbs and natural ingredients. Whether it's a soothing tea to enhance sleep quality, a potent herbal tincture to reduce inflammation, or a nutrient-dense meal to support robust health, each entry is crafted with the goal of advancing your understanding and implementation of effective natural health practices.

Let's embark on this journey of discovery, where each recipe and remedy is a step towards optimizing your health and extending your years of active, vibrant living.

ANTI-INFLAMMATORY REMEDIES

1. Turmeric and Black Pepper Capsules

Description:

Combines the potent anti-inflammatory properties of curcumin from turmeric with piperine from black pepper for enhanced absorption and effectiveness.

Ingredients:

- Turmeric powder
- Black pepper powder
- Empty capsules

Preparation Steps:

1. Combine two parts turmeric powder with one part black pepper powder to increase curcumin absorption.
2. Carefully open the empty capsules and fill them with the turmeric and black pepper mixture, packing the powder tightly.
3. Close the capsules, using a capsule filling machine if available.
4. Store the filled capsules in a cool, dry place, ideally in a glass jar with a tight lid to keep moisture out.

Usage:

Take one capsule with meals, up to three times per day, or as directed by a healthcare provider.

Benefits:

Regular consumption of these capsules can manage and reduce inflammation, relieve joint pain and stiffness, and support overall health by improving liver function, aiding digestion, and boosting immune health.

2. Ginger Tea

Description:

Fresh ginger steeped in hot water, effective at reducing inflammation and soothing digestive issues.

Ingredients:

- Fresh ginger root
- Hot water

Preparation Steps:

1. Slice a 1-inch piece of fresh ginger root.
2. Steep the ginger slices in a cup of hot water for about 10 minutes.
3. Strain the ginger pieces from the water before drinking.

Usage:

Drink a cup of ginger tea twice daily, especially before meals to aid digestion or whenever experiencing digestive discomfort.

Benefits:

Ginger tea is not only comforting but also beneficial for its anti-inflammatory properties that can help reduce pain and promote digestive health. Regular consumption can ease stomach discomfort and support overall digestive function.

3. Omega-3 Fish Oil Supplements

Description:

High in EPA and DHA, these supplements are crucial for reducing systemic inflammation.

Usage:

Take one to two capsules daily, preferably with meals to improve absorption and reduce the risk of digestive discomfort.

Benefits:

Omega-3 supplements are essential for their powerful anti-inflammatory effects, which can benefit cardiovascular health, cognitive function, and joint mobility. Regular intake helps maintain a healthy inflammatory response throughout the body.

4. Green Tea Extract

Description:

Rich in polyphenols like EGCG, which have significant anti-inflammatory properties.

Usage:

Consume one capsule daily or as recommended on the supplement label, preferably with a meal to enhance absorption.

Benefits:

Green tea extract is beneficial for reducing inflammation due to its high content of antioxidant polyphenols. Regular consumption can aid in protecting against oxidative stress and supporting overall cellular health.

5. Cherry Juice

Description:

Contains anthocyanins that help reduce inflammation and muscle soreness, particularly beneficial for athletes.

Usage:

Drink 8-10 ounces of cherry juice twice a day,

ideally post-exercise or before bedtime to aid recovery and reduce soreness.

Benefits:

Cherry juice is renowned for its ability to combat inflammation and accelerate muscle recovery. Its high antioxidant content not only alleviates muscle soreness but also supports overall joint and cardiovascular health.

6. Maritime Pine Bark Extract

Description:

Pycnogenol®, derived from maritime pine bark, is known for its potent antioxidative and anti-inflammatory properties.

Usage:

Take one capsule daily, or as recommended on the supplement packaging, preferably with a meal to optimize absorption.

Benefits:

Maritime pine bark extract helps reduce oxidative stress and inflammation, supporting vascular health and enhancing skin elasticity. Its broad antioxidant effects are beneficial for overall cellular health and longevity.

7. Flaxseed Smoothie

Description:

Ground flaxseeds mixed into a smoothie provide ALA, a plant-based omega-3 fatty acid that combats inflammation.

Ingredients:

- Ground flaxseeds
- Your choice of milk (dairy or plant-based)
- Optional: fruits, vegetables, and other smoothie additives

Preparation Steps:

1. Measure one to two tablespoons of ground flaxseeds.
2. Blend the ground flaxseeds with one cup of your preferred milk and any additional fruits or vegetables for flavor and added nutrients.
3. Blend until smooth.

Usage:

Enjoy this flaxseed smoothie once daily, preferably in the morning or as a post-workout meal to maximize its anti-inflammatory benefits.

Benefits:

The ALA in flaxseeds helps reduce inflammation throughout the body, supporting cardiovascular health and overall well-being. Incorporating this smoothie into your daily routine can also aid in digestion and enhance nutrient absorption.

8. CBD Oil

Description:

Cannabidiol (CBD) oil is derived from the cannabis plant and has been shown to help reduce chronic pain and inflammation without psychoactive effects.

Ingredients:

CBD oil (full-spectrum or broad-spectrum recommended)

Usage:

Administer a few drops of CBD oil under the tongue once or twice daily, or as directed by the packaging. Hold the oil under the tongue for 30-60 seconds before swallowing for optimal absorption.

Benefits:

CBD oil is effective in managing chronic pain, reducing inflammation, and improving sleep quality without the intoxicating effects associated with THC. Regular use can contribute to improved joint mobility and overall stress reduction, enhancing quality of life.

9. Aloe Vera Juice

Description:

Aloe vera juice is taken internally for its anti-inflammatory and digestive soothing properties, promoting gut health and reducing inflammation.

Usage:

Drink 2 to 4 ounces of aloe vera juice daily, either alone or mixed with water or another juice to enhance palatability. It's best consumed on an empty stomach to maximize absorption and effectiveness.

Benefits:

Aloe vera juice helps soothe the lining of the stomach and intestines, reducing gastrointestinal inflammation and promoting healing. Regular consumption can aid in improving digestion, maintaining hydration, and supporting nutrient absorption.

10. Boswellia Tablets

Description:

Boswellia, also known as Indian Frankincense, is used in tablet form for its effectiveness in reducing inflammation associated with arthritis and other chronic inflammatory conditions.

Usage:

Take one Boswellia tablet per the dosage instructions on the package, typically one to three times daily with food to minimize potential digestive upset.

Benefits:

Boswellia is renowned for its powerful anti-inflammatory effects, particularly in reducing pain and swelling in arthritis sufferers. Regular use can

enhance joint function and mobility, contributing to improved overall quality of life in individuals dealing with chronic inflammatory conditions.

11. Moringa Leaf Powder

Description:

Moringa leaf powder is packed with natural anti-inflammatory compounds and can be easily added to smoothies, teas, or other dishes for health enhancement.

Usage:

Incorporate a teaspoon of moringa leaf powder into your daily diet by adding it to a morning smoothie, mixing it into a cup of warm tea, or sprinkling it over meals.

Benefits:

Moringa is celebrated for its comprehensive health benefits, including reducing inflammation, boosting antioxidant levels, and enhancing energy. Its high nutrient density supports overall health and helps in managing symptoms of inflammation-based conditions.

12. Tart Cherry Extract Capsules

Description:

Tart cherry extract is known for its effectiveness in reducing inflammation and aiding muscle recovery, making it particularly valued by athletes and those with chronic joint pain.

Ingredients:

- Tart cherry powder
- Empty capsules

Preparation Steps:

1. Purchase high-quality tart cherry powder, ensuring it contains a high concentration of anthocyanins for maximum effectiveness.

2. If using a capsule filling machine, set it up according to the manufacturer's instructions. Place the larger half of the capsules in the base of the machine.

3. Distribute the tart cherry powder evenly into the capsule bases. If not using a machine, manually fill each capsule half with the measured amount of powder.

4. Seal the capsules by placing the smaller half on top and pressing down to close them securely.

5. Store the filled capsules in a cool, dry place, ideally in a dark container to protect from light.

6. Alternatively, pre-made tart cherry extract capsules are available for purchase if you prefer a ready-to-use option without the need for DIY preparation.

Usage:

Consume one capsule of tart cherry extract one to two times daily, with or without food. It is especially beneficial when taken post-exercise to aid recovery or before bedtime to improve sleep quality.

Benefits:

Regular consumption of tart cherry extract capsules helps reduce inflammation and muscle soreness after physical activities. The natural anti-inflammatory and antioxidant properties support overall health and recovery, making it an excellent supplement for enhancing physical performance and well-being.

13. Spirulina

Description:

Spirulina, a blue-green algae, is renowned for its ability to reduce inflammation and boost antioxidant protection, making it a popular supplement for enhancing overall health.

Ingredients:

1. Spirulina powder

2. Empty capsules (for DIY capsule making)

Preparation Steps:

1. Purchase high-quality, pure spirulina powder, ensuring it is free from contaminants and additives for optimal health benefits.

2. For DIY capsules: Using a capsule filling machine, place the larger half of the capsules in the base. Evenly distribute the spirulina powder into the capsule bases. If not using a machine, manually fill each capsule half with the measured amount of spirulina. Seal the capsules by placing the smaller half on top and pressing down to close them securely. Store the filled capsules in a cool, dry place, ideally in a dark container to protect from light.

3. Alternatively, pre-made spirulina capsules are available for purchase if you prefer a ready-to-use option without the need for DIY preparation.

Usage:

Consume one spirulina capsule one to two times daily, preferably with meals to aid digestion and absorption.

Benefits:

Spirulina is highly effective in reducing systemic inflammation and enhancing the body's antioxidant defenses. Its rich nutrient profile supports immune health, promotes energy levels, and aids in detoxification, contributing to overall vitality and well-being.

14. Rosehip Tea

Description:

Rosehip tea, made from the fruit of the rose plant, is valued for its polyphenols and galactolipids, which offer significant anti-inflammatory effects.

Ingredients:

□ Dried rosehips

▫ Hot water

Preparation Steps:

1. Purchase high-quality, organic dried rosehips to ensure they are free from pesticides and other contaminants.

2. To make the tea, measure about one tablespoon of dried rosehips.

3. Steep the dried rosehips in a cup of boiling water for 10-15 minutes to fully extract the beneficial compounds.

4. Strain the tea to remove the rosehips before drinking.

5. Alternatively, pre-packaged rosehip tea bags are available for those who prefer convenience without the need for DIY preparation.

Usage:

Drink rosehip tea once or twice daily. Enjoying a cup in the morning can kickstart your day with anti-inflammatory benefits, or sip it in the evening to unwind.

Benefits:

Regular consumption of rosehip tea helps reduce inflammation throughout the body, particularly beneficial for joint health and reducing symptoms of arthritis. The tea's high vitamin C content also supports immune health and skin rejuvenation, making it a nourishing choice for overall well-being.

15. Resveratrol Supplements

Description:

Resveratrol, a potent compound found in the skin of red grapes, supports health and longevity through its strong anti-inflammatory actions.

Usage:

Take one resveratrol supplement daily, preferably with food to enhance absorption and maximize its anti-inflammatory benefits.

Benefits:

Regular intake of resveratrol supplements can significantly reduce inflammation, potentially lowering the risk of chronic diseases such as heart disease and certain cancers. Its antioxidant properties also help protect cells from damage, supporting overall health and aging well.

16. Licorice Root Tea

Description:

Licorice root tea, infused with the active compound glycyrrhizin, helps reduce inflammation and soothe gastrointestinal issues, making it a beneficial drink for digestive health.

Ingredients:

Dried licorice root

Hot water

Preparation Steps:

1. Select high-quality, organic dried licorice root to ensure purity and effectiveness.

2. Measure about one teaspoon of dried licorice root.

3. Steep the licorice root in a cup of boiling water for 10-15 minutes to fully extract the glycyrrhizin and other beneficial compounds.

4. Strain the tea to remove the licorice pieces before drinking.

5. For those who prefer convenience, pre-packaged licorice root tea bags are also available and eliminate the need for DIY preparation.

Usage:

Drink licorice root tea once or twice daily, particularly before meals to aid digestion or whenever experiencing stomach discomfort.

Benefits:

Licorice root tea is particularly effective in soothing the stomach, reducing inflammation in the digestive tract, and supporting overall gastrointestinal health. Its anti-inflammatory properties also contribute to immune system support and can help manage symptoms of chronic inflammatory conditions.

17. Fermented Papaya Concentrate

Description:

Fermented papaya concentrate is celebrated for its anti-inflammatory properties and its ability to aid digestion, making it a valuable supplement for gut health.

Usage:

Consume a small amount of papaya concentrate, about one tablespoon, daily either directly or mixed into water or juice.

Benefits:

Regular consumption helps reduce systemic inflammation and improves digestive efficiency, supporting overall wellness and nutrient absorption.

18. White Willow Bark Capsules

Description:

White willow bark, the natural precursor to aspirin, is utilized for its pain relief and anti-inflammatory properties, making it a natural alternative for managing discomfort.

Ingredients:

- White willow bark powder
- Empty capsules

Preparation Steps:

1. Source high-quality, pure white willow bark powder, ensuring it is free from contaminants and additives.

2. If preparing capsules, use a capsule filling machine to fill empty capsules with measured amounts of white willow bark powder. Seal the capsules securely.

3. Store the filled capsules in a cool, dry place, away from direct sunlight to maintain potency.

4. Pre-made white willow bark capsules are also available for those seeking convenience without the DIY process.

Usage:

Take one capsule of white willow bark, typically 1-2 times per day, as needed for pain or as directed by a healthcare provider.

Benefits:

White willow bark provides effective pain relief and reduces inflammation, making it beneficial for treating headaches, muscle pain, and joint discomfort.

19. Matcha Green Tea

Description:

Matcha green tea, concentrated and higher in antioxidants than regular green tea, aids in fighting inflammation and enhancing overall health.

Ingredients:

- Matcha green tea powder
- Hot water

Preparation Steps:

1. Choose ceremonial-grade matcha green tea powder for the highest quality and antioxidant content.

2. Sift about one teaspoon of matcha powder into a bowl to remove any clumps.

3. Add hot water (not boiling) to the bowl and whisk vigorously until the tea becomes frothy.

4. For convenience, pre-packaged matcha tea bags are available, though they may contain less matcha than using the powder directly.

Usage:

Enjoy a cup of matcha green tea daily, preferably in the morning to benefit from its energizing properties without disrupting sleep.

Benefits:

Regular consumption of matcha boosts antioxidant intake, helping to reduce cellular damage and inflammation, supporting cardiovascular health and enhancing overall wellness.

20. Bromelain Supplements

Description:

Bromelain, an enzyme extracted from pineapple, is recognized for its effectiveness in treating inflammation and aiding digestion.

Usage:

Take bromelain according to the dosage instructions on the package, typically one to two capsules daily, with or between meals, depending on whether you're using it for digestive aid or inflammation.

Benefits:

Bromelain supplements help reduce inflammation and improve digestion, offering relief from conditions like sinusitis, arthritis, and digestive disorders.

21. Ashwagandha Root Extract

Description:

Ashwagandha root extract is an adaptogen known for its ability to help the body manage stress and combat inflammation, enhancing overall wellness.

Usage:

Take ashwagandha root extract as directed on the packaging, generally one to two times daily, preferably with meals to support absorption and reduce the potential for stomach upset.

Benefits:

Regular intake of ashwagandha root extract can significantly enhance the body's stress response, reduce inflammation, and support immune function, contributing to improved vitality and better stress management.

22. Nettle Leaf Tea

Description:

Nettle leaf tea is recognized for its natural antihistamine properties, making it an effective remedy for allergic inflammation and related symptoms.

Ingredients:

☐ Dried nettle leaves

☐ Hot water

Preparation Steps:

1. Choose high-quality, organic dried nettle leaves to ensure purity and effectiveness.

2. Steep about one tablespoon of dried nettle leaves in a cup of boiling water for 10-15 minutes to fully extract the beneficial compounds.

3. Strain the leaves from the tea before drinking.

4. Alternatively, pre-packaged nettle leaf tea bags are available for those who prefer a more convenient option without the need for loose leaves.

Usage:

Drink nettle leaf tea once or twice daily, especially

during allergy seasons, to maximize its anti-inflammatory and antihistamine effects.

Benefits:

Regular consumption of nettle leaf tea can help alleviate symptoms of allergies such as sneezing, itchy eyes, and nasal congestion. Its natural anti-inflammatory properties also support overall immune health.

23. Golden Milk Powder

Description:

Golden Milk Powder is a blend of turmeric, ginger, and cinnamon, designed to create a soothing, anti-inflammatory drink that promotes relaxation and wellness.

Ingredients:

- Turmeric powder
- Ginger powder
- Cinnamon powder
- Black pepper (to enhance turmeric absorption)

Preparation Steps:

1. Combine equal parts of turmeric, ginger, and cinnamon powders. Add a small amount of black pepper to the mix to increase the bioavailability of curcumin from turmeric.

2. Mix the ingredients thoroughly and store in an airtight container in a cool, dry place.

3. Pre-made Golden Milk Powder is also available for purchase if you prefer convenience and consistency in your blends.

Usage:

To make Golden Milk, mix one teaspoon of Golden Milk Powder with a cup of warm milk (dairy or plant-based). Stir well and add a sweetener if desired, such as honey or maple syrup. Drink this mixture once a day, preferably before bedtime, to maximize its soothing effects.

Benefits:

Golden Milk made from this powder helps reduce inflammation, supports digestive health, and boosts the immune system. The spices in this blend are also known for their antioxidant properties, contributing to overall health and well-being.

24. Saffron Threads

Description:

Saffron threads are celebrated for their potent antioxidant properties, which help reduce inflammation and promote overall wellness.

For use, a small quantity is typically sufficient due to its strong flavor and high potency.

Usage:

Add a few strands of saffron to warm water or milk and let it steep for 5 to 10 minutes to release its flavor and beneficial compounds. Drink this infusion once daily, or use saffron in cooking to enhance dishes while gaining its health benefits.

Benefits:

Regular consumption of saffron can help alleviate symptoms of inflammation and enhance mood. Its antioxidant capabilities support cellular health and can contribute to a reduction in stress and anxiety levels.

25. Curry Leaf Infusion

Description:

Curry leaf infusion is utilized for its anti-inflammatory properties, particularly effective in combating inflammation in the joints and muscles.

Ingredients:

- Fresh or dried curry leaves

Preparation Steps:

1. Choose fresh or high-quality dried curry leaves. If using fresh leaves, ensure they are clean and free from any pesticides.

2. For a simple infusion, steep about 10-15 curry leaves in a cup of boiling water for 8-10 minutes.

3. Strain the leaves out before drinking.

4. Store any unused dried curry leaves in a cool, dry place in an airtight container to maintain freshness.

Usage:

Drink a cup of curry leaf infusion once daily, especially after physical activities or during times of increased joint or muscle discomfort.

Benefits:

Regular consumption of curry leaf infusion can significantly reduce inflammation in the body, offering relief from joint pain and muscle soreness. Its natural anti-inflammatory properties also support overall health and well-being.

DIGESTIVE HEALTH REMEDIES

26. Probiotic Yogurt

Description:

Probiotic yogurt is enriched with live beneficial bacteria that help maintain a healthy gut microbiome, essential for optimal digestive health.

Usage:

Incorporate one cup of probiotic yogurt into your daily diet. It can be consumed on its own or mixed with fruits, nuts, or honey to enhance its flavor and nutritional value.

Benefits:

Regular consumption of probiotic yogurt supports digestive health by promoting a balanced gut flora. This not only aids in digestion and nutrient absorption but also boosts the immune system and helps prevent common gastrointestinal issues such as bloating and diarrhea.

27. Ginger Digestive Chews

Description:

Ginger Digestive Chews harness the natural properties of ginger to ease nausea, improve digestion, and reduce bloating, offering a convenient and tasty way to benefit from ginger's medicinal qualities.

Ingredients:

- Fresh ginger
- Sugar or honey
- Optional flavorings (e.g., lemon zest, mint)

Preparation Steps:

1. Peel and grate a fresh ginger root.

2. In a saucepan, combine the grated ginger with sugar or honey and a little water. Cook over low heat until the mixture thickens.

3. If desired, add optional flavorings like lemon zest or mint for enhanced taste.

4. Allow the mixture to cool slightly, then form it into small chew-sized pieces. Roll them in a coating of sugar if desired and let them harden on parchment paper.

Usage:

Consume one or two ginger chews daily, especially before or after meals, to aid digestion or whenever experiencing stomach discomfort or nausea.

Benefits:

Ginger chews offer a practical and enjoyable way to utilize ginger's anti-inflammatory and gastrointestinal soothing properties, aiding in digestion, reducing nausea, and minimizing bloating.

28. Peppermint Oil

Capsules

Description:

Peppermint oil capsules are often used to relieve symptoms of Irritable Bowel Syndrome (IBS) and soothe digestive spasms, leveraging peppermint's natural antispasmodic and soothing properties.

Usage:

Take one peppermint oil capsule one to three times daily, preferably before meals to optimize digestive comfort and effectiveness.

Benefits:

Peppermint oil capsules effectively reduce gastrointestinal discomfort by relaxing the smooth muscles of the gastrointestinal tract. This action helps alleviate symptoms of IBS, including bloating, gas, and intermittent abdominal pain, promoting a smoother digestive process.

29. Fennel Seed Tea

Description:

Fennel seed tea is renowned for its ability to relax the gastrointestinal tract and reduce symptoms of gas and bloating, making it a beneficial drink for digestive wellness.

Ingredients:

- Fennel seeds
- Hot water

Preparation Steps:

1. Crush a teaspoon of fennel seeds to release their oils and potent flavor.

2. Steep the crushed seeds in a cup of boiling water for 5-10 minutes.

3. Strain the seeds from the water before drinking.

Usage:

Drink a cup of fennel seed tea after meals or when experiencing digestive discomfort to harness its soothing effects.

Benefits:

Regular consumption of fennel seed tea can significantly ease digestive spasms, reduce bloating and gas, and promote overall digestive health, enhancing comfort and nutrient absorption.

30. Apple Cider Vinegar Tonic

Description:

Apple cider vinegar tonic is taken before meals to enhance digestive enzymes and balance stomach acid, aiding in improved digestion and nutrient absorption.

Ingredients:

- Apple cider vinegar
- Water
- Optional: honey or lemon for flavor

Preparation Steps:

1. Dilute one to two tablespoons of apple cider vinegar in a glass of water.

2. Add honey or lemon to taste, if desired, to improve the flavor of the tonic.

Usage:

Drink this tonic about 20-30 minutes before meals to prepare the digestive system for food intake.

Benefits:

Apple cider vinegar tonic can help stimulate digestive juices, leading to better breakdown and absorption of nutrients. It also helps in maintaining a healthy pH balance in the stomach, which can alleviate common digestive discomforts like heartburn and indigestion.

31. Inulin Fiber Supplement

Description:

Inulin fiber supplement acts as a prebiotic, feeding beneficial gut bacteria and supporting overall digestive health by enhancing gut flora balance.

Usage:

Take an inulin fiber supplement according to the dosage instructions on the package, typically mixed into a glass of water or added to foods such as yogurt or smoothies. It is best consumed with meals to facilitate digestion and the absorption of nutrients.

Benefits:

Regular intake of inulin fiber promotes the growth of beneficial gut bacteria, which plays a crucial role in digestion, nutrient absorption, and immune function. This supplementation can help maintain healthy digestion, reduce bloating, and prevent constipation, contributing to better gastrointestinal health and comfort.

32. Dandelion Root Tea

Description:

Dandelion root tea is known for stimulating digestion and supporting liver detoxification, making it a beneficial herbal tea for enhancing metabolic health.

Ingredients:

- Dried dandelion root
- Hot water

Preparation Steps:

1. Steep one to two teaspoons of dried dandelion root in a cup of boiling water for 10-15 minutes.
2. Strain the roots from the tea before drinking.

Usage:

Drink a cup of dandelion root tea daily, preferably before meals to stimulate digestive enzymes and support liver health.

Benefits:

Regular consumption of dandelion root tea helps enhance digestive function and supports the liver in detoxifying the body. Its natural diuretic properties also contribute to detoxification, promoting overall health and well-being.

33. Kefir

Description:

Kefir is a fermented milk drink rich in probiotics, known for its extensive benefits for gut health and overall wellness.

Ingredients:

- Milk (dairy or non-dairy alternatives like coconut milk)
- Kefir grains

Preparation Steps:

1. Mix kefir grains with milk in a clean glass jar.
2. Cover the jar with a breathable cloth secured with a rubber band, allowing for air circulation while keeping contaminants out.
3. Let the mixture ferment at room temperature for 24 to 48 hours until the milk thickens and takes on a tangy flavor.
4. Strain out the kefir grains. These can be reused for subsequent batches.
5. Store the finished kefir in the refrigerator.

Usage:

Consume a glass of kefir daily, either on its own or blended into smoothies, to support digestive health and boost immunity.

Benefits:

Regular consumption of kefir significantly enhances the gut microbiota with its diverse range of beneficial bacteria and yeasts, improving digestion and nutrient absorption. The probiotics in kefir also strengthen the immune system and can help maintain overall health.

34. Digestive Enzyme Supplements

Description:

Digestive enzyme supplements assist in the breakdown of fats, proteins, and carbohydrates, enhancing nutrient absorption and improving overall digestive efficiency.

Usage:

Take a digestive enzyme supplement just before or during each meal, following the dosage recommendations on the product packaging. This timing ensures the enzymes are available when needed to aid in the digestion of food.

Benefits:

Regular use of digestive enzyme supplements can significantly reduce digestive discomforts such as bloating, gas, and feelings of fullness after meals. By enhancing the breakdown and absorption of nutrients, these supplements support optimal nutrition and contribute to overall gastrointestinal health.

35. Slippery Elm Bark Powder

Description:

Slippery elm bark powder is known for forming a soothing film over the digestive tract, helping alleviate issues such as acid reflux and ulcers.

Ingredients:

□ Slippery elm bark powder

□ Hot water

Preparation Steps:

1. Mix one to two teaspoons of slippery elm bark powder with hot water to create a smooth, gel-like consistency.

2. Stir thoroughly until the powder is fully dissolved.

Usage:

Drink the slippery elm mixture once or twice daily, preferably between meals or at bedtime to maximize its soothing effects on the digestive tract.

Benefits:

Slippery elm bark powder forms a protective layer on the lining of the digestive tract, which helps soothe irritation, reduce inflammation, and promote healing of ulcers and acid reflux symptoms. This natural demulcent is particularly beneficial for those with sensitive digestive systems.

36. Chamomile Tea

Description:

Chamomile tea is celebrated for its soothing effects that help relax the gastrointestinal muscles and reduce discomfort, making it an ideal herbal tea for digestive health.

Ingredients:

□ Dried chamomile flowers

□ Hot water

Preparation Steps:

1. Steep one to two teaspoons of dried chamomile flowers in a cup of boiling water for 5-10 minutes.

2. Strain the flowers to remove them from the tea.

Usage:

Drink a cup of chamomile tea in the evening or after meals to benefit from its calming effects on the digestive system.

Benefits:

Regular consumption of chamomile tea helps soothe the digestive tract, alleviating symptoms of indigestion, gas, and bloating. Its mild sedative properties also contribute to stress reduction and improved sleep quality, further enhancing digestive health.

37. Bone Broth

Description:

Bone broth is rich in collagen and amino acids, essential for healing and strengthening the gut lining, supporting overall digestive health.

Ingredients:

- Bones (chicken, beef, or fish)
- Water
- Acidic component (vinegar or lemon juice)
- Optional: vegetables and herbs for flavor

Preparation Steps:

1. Place bones in a large pot or slow cooker and cover with water. Add a splash of vinegar or lemon juice to help extract nutrients from the bones.

2. Bring to a boil, then reduce heat to simmer. Optionally, add vegetables like carrots, onions, and celery, and herbs such as thyme and bay leaves for enhanced flavor.

3. Simmer for 12-24 hours, skimming off any foam that forms on the surface.

4. Strain the broth through a fine mesh sieve to remove solids.

Usage:

Consume a cup of bone broth daily, either as a warm drink or incorporated into soups and stews, to utilize its gut-healing benefits.

Benefits:

Regular intake of bone broth promotes a healthy digestive system by providing collagen and amino acids that repair and strengthen the gut lining. Its anti-inflammatory properties also aid in reducing gastrointestinal inflammation, supporting overall digestive function.

38. Lacto-Fermented Vegetables

Description:

Lacto-fermented vegetables, such as sauerkraut and kimchi, are rich in live probiotics and enzymes that boost digestive health and enhance gut flora.

Ingredients:

- Fresh vegetables (cabbage for sauerkraut, a mix of cabbage and other vegetables for kimchi)
- Salt
- Water
- Optional: spices and other flavorings (garlic, ginger, chili peppers for kimchi)

Preparation Steps:

1. Chop or shred the chosen vegetables.

2. For sauerkraut, mix the shredded cabbage with salt and pack it tightly into a clean jar, letting the salt draw out the water to create brine.

3. For kimchi, mix the vegetables with salt and spices, then pack into a jar and cover with water if needed to submerge the vegetables.

4. Ensure the vegetables are fully submerged under the brine to prevent mold. Cover the jar with a cloth or a lid that allows gases to escape.

5. Leave the jar at room temperature for several days, checking regularly and pressing down the vegetables if they rise above the brine.

6. Once fermented, store in the refrigerator to slow down the fermentation process.

Usage:

Incorporate lacto-fermented vegetables into your daily meals, eating a small amount with each meal to aid digestion and introduce beneficial probiotics into your diet.

Benefits:

Regular consumption of lacto-fermented vegetables like sauerkraut and kimchi introduces beneficial probiotics that support the digestive system, enhance nutrient absorption, and strengthen the immune system. The fermentation process also increases the bioavailability of nutrients, making these vegetables a powerhouse for digestive health.

39. Activated Charcoal Capsules

Description:

Activated charcoal capsules are used occasionally to bind toxins and assist with digestion, especially useful during dietary indiscretions or after consuming questionable foods.

Ingredients:

- Activated charcoal powder
- Empty capsules

Preparation Steps:

1. Purchase high-quality activated charcoal powder.

2. If filling your own capsules, use a capsule filling machine to fill empty capsules with the charcoal powder. Ensure a tight seal to prevent any leakage.

3. Store the filled capsules in a cool, dry place to maintain potency.

4. Alternatively, pre-made activated charcoal capsules are available for those seeking convenience without the DIY process.

Usage:

Take one to two activated charcoal capsules as needed, ideally within an hour after consuming suspect foods or during digestive upset. It's important to use them only on occasion and not as a regular supplement.

Benefits:

Activated charcoal is highly absorbent, helping to bind and remove toxins and gases from the digestive system, which can alleviate bloating and discomfort following dietary mishaps. Its use can also help prevent the systemic absorption of unwanted substances from the gut.

40. Artichoke Leaf Extract

Description:

Artichoke leaf extract stimulates bile production, enhancing fat digestion and liver health, making it a valuable supplement for improving digestive efficiency.

Usage:

Take one artichoke leaf extract capsule with meals, particularly with high-fat foods, to enhance bile production and support digestion.

Benefits:

Regular intake of artichoke leaf extract can improve bile flow, which is essential for the digestion and absorption of fats, and promote liver health. This helps to alleviate symptoms such as bloating and indigestion after eating fatty meals, and supports overall digestive function.

41. Licorice Root Deglycyrrhizinated (DGL)

Description:

Licorice Root Deglycyrrhizinated (DGL) is specially processed to remove glycyrrhizin, reducing the risk of high blood pressure while retaining its ability to soothe gastrointestinal inflammation and protect against ulcer formation.

Usage:

Chew one DGL tablet or take as directed 20-30 minutes before meals to maximize its protective and soothing effects on the gastrointestinal tract.

Benefits:

Regular use of DGL licorice helps soothe and protect the digestive lining, effectively reducing inflammation and preventing the development of ulcers. Its action supports a healthy stomach lining while avoiding the side effects associated with traditional licorice root, making it suitable for regular use.

42. Aloe Vera Juice

Description:

Aloe vera juice is celebrated for its natural healing and soothing properties, particularly effective for the digestive tract, helping to heal irritated or inflamed mucosal linings.

Usage:

Drink a small glass (about 2-4 ounces) of aloe vera juice daily, either on its own or diluted in water or another juice to improve taste and digestion.

Benefits:

Aloe vera juice helps soothe the lining of the digestive tract, reducing symptoms of conditions like acid reflux, gastritis, and ulcers. Its anti-inflammatory properties also aid in healing and maintaining a healthy gut, promoting overall digestive wellness.

43. Psyllium Husk

Description:

Psyllium husk is a fiber supplement known for

helping maintain bowel regularity and promoting satiety, making it an effective aid for digestive health and weight management.

Usage:

Mix one to two teaspoons of psyllium husk powder in a glass of water or your preferred beverage and drink immediately before it thickens. If using capsules, follow the dosage instructions provided on the package. It's important to consume psyllium with sufficient water to facilitate its digestive benefits.

Benefits:

Regular intake of psyllium husk enhances digestive regularity by increasing stool bulk and promoting a natural, healthy bowel movement cycle. Its high fiber content also helps control hunger and maintain a healthy weight by promoting a feeling of fullness.

44. Triphala Powder

Description:

Triphala powder is an Ayurvedic blend of three fruits—Amalaki, Bibhitaki, and Haritaki—that tones the gut, supports regular bowel movements, and aids in detoxification, enhancing overall digestive health.

Usage:

Mix about one-half to one teaspoon of Triphala powder in a glass of warm water and drink it on an empty stomach at bedtime or upon waking.

Benefits:

Regular use of Triphala powder helps maintain digestive balance by promoting regular bowel movements and cleansing the digestive tract. Its natural antioxidant properties also support detoxification and contribute to improved gut health and overall vitality.

45. Mint Leaf Capsules

Description:

Mint leaf capsules offer relief from indigestion and symptoms of irritable bowel syndrome (IBS), harnessing the soothing properties of mint to improve digestive wellness.

Usage:

Take one mint leaf capsule with water, usually before meals or at the onset of indigestion or IBS symptoms, as directed on the package.

Benefits:

Mint leaf capsules effectively alleviate digestive issues such as bloating, gas, and discomfort associated with indigestion and IBS. Their natural antispasmodic properties help relax the digestive tract muscles, providing symptomatic relief and enhancing digestive function.

46. Senna Tea

Description:

Senna tea acts as a natural laxative, effectively used for relieving occasional constipation. Its compounds stimulate bowel movements, making it a quick-acting solution for digestive discomfort.

Ingredients:

- Dried senna leaves
- Hot water

Preparation Steps:

1. Steep one to two teaspoons of dried senna leaves in a cup of boiling water for 5-10 minutes.

2. Strain the leaves out before drinking the tea to ensure proper dosage and to avoid consuming leaf particles.

3. Pre-packaged senna tea bags are also available, providing a convenient and precisely dosed option.

Usage:

Drink one cup of senna tea at bedtime or as

needed for constipation relief. Do not use senna tea for more than 7-10 consecutive days without consulting a healthcare provider to avoid dependency.

Benefits:

Senna tea is effective for short-term relief of constipation, promoting regular bowel movements and helping to cleanse the colon. Its natural laxative properties facilitate easier stool passage and can aid in detoxifying the digestive system.

47. Papaya Enzyme Chewables

Description:

Papaya enzyme chewables contain papain, a potent enzyme that helps digest proteins and soothes the stomach, making them an excellent aid for improving digestion and reducing discomfort after meals.

Usage:

Chew one papaya enzyme tablet immediately after meals or when experiencing digestive discomfort, such as bloating or indigestion.

Benefits:

Regular use of papaya enzyme chewables can significantly aid in the digestion of proteins, reduce bloating, and alleviate symptoms of indigestion. Their soothing effect on the stomach helps to maintain a comfortable and efficient digestive process.

48. Lemon Balm Tea

Description:

Lemon balm tea is known for easing abdominal pain and discomfort associated with digestion, offering a soothing remedy for the gastrointestinal tract.

Ingredients:

- Dried lemon balm leaves
- Hot water

Preparation Steps:

1. Steep one to two teaspoons of dried lemon balm leaves in a cup of boiling water for 5-10 minutes.

2. Strain the leaves to remove them before drinking.

3. Pre-packaged lemon balm tea bags are also available, providing a convenient way to enjoy this herbal remedy without preparation.

Usage:

Drink lemon balm tea one to two times daily, particularly after meals or whenever experiencing digestive discomfort, to benefit from its calming effects.

Benefits:

Regular consumption of lemon balm tea can help relieve symptoms of indigestion such as gas, bloating, and abdominal pain. Its mild sedative properties also contribute to relaxation and can aid in reducing stress, further alleviating digestive issues.

49. Bitter Greens Supplement

Description:

Bitter greens supplements contain a blend of bitter herbs known to stimulate digestive juices and support liver function, enhancing digestion and overall detoxification processes.

Usage:

Take one bitter greens supplement daily, preferably before meals, to stimulate digestive enzymes and support liver health.

Benefits:

Regular intake of bitter greens supplements aids in digestion by promoting the production of digestive enzymes and enhancing bile flow. This not only helps in breaking down fats but also supports liver detoxification, contributing to improved metabolic health and nutrient absorption.

50. Bacillus Coagulans Probiotic

Description:

Bacillus coagulans is a resilient probiotic that survives stomach acid, making it exceptionally effective in supporting gut health and enhancing the intestinal flora.

Usage:

Take one Bacillus coagulans probiotic capsule daily, preferably with a meal, to enhance its survival through the digestive tract and maximize its benefits.

Benefits:

Regular use of Bacillus coagulans probiotics supports a healthy digestive system by maintaining a balanced gut microbiome, which is crucial for effective digestion, nutrient absorption, and immune function. Its ability to survive stomach acid ensures that it reaches the intestines where it can have the most impact, helping to prevent and alleviate common gastrointestinal disorders such as bloating and irregularity.

IMMUNE SUPPORT REMEDIES

51. Elderberry Syrup

Description:

Elderberry syrup is rich in antioxidants and vitamins, recognized for its ability to help prevent and ease cold and flu symptoms, making it a staple in natural immune support.

Ingredients:

- Elderberries
- Water
- Honey or another natural sweetener

Preparation Steps:

1. Simmer fresh or dried elderberries in water for about 45 minutes to extract their juice and nutrients.
2. Strain the mixture to remove the solids and add honey to the liquid while still warm to sweeten and enhance the syrup's preserving properties.
3. Store the finished syrup in a glass bottle in the refrigerator to maintain its potency.
4. Alternatively, pre-made elderberry syrup is available for those seeking convenience without the need for DIY preparation.

Usage:

Take one tablespoon of elderberry syrup daily during cold and flu season to boost immunity, or every few hours when experiencing acute cold or flu symptoms.

Benefits:

Elderberry syrup provides significant immune support, thanks to its high levels of vitamins A, B, and C, and antioxidants. Regular consumption can help reduce the duration and severity of cold and flu symptoms, support respiratory health, and strengthen the immune system.

52. Vitamin C Boosting Smoothie

Description:

This Vitamin C boosting smoothie combines citrus fruits, kiwi, and strawberries, all known for their high vitamin C content, which is crucial for enhancing immune function and overall health.

Ingredients:

- Oranges
- Kiwis
- Strawberries
- Optional: a splash of water or orange juice for easier blending

Preparation Steps:

1. Peel and segment oranges, peel and slice kiwis, and hull strawberries.
2. Place all fruits in a blender, adding a small amount of water or orange juice if needed to facilitate blending.
3. Blend until smooth.
4. Pour into a glass and enjoy immediately to ensure maximum nutrient intake.

Usage:

Drink this Vitamin C boosting smoothie daily, particularly during cold and flu season or whenever extra immune support is needed.

Benefits:

Rich in Vitamin C, this smoothie supports the immune system, reduces oxidative stress, and enhances the body's ability to fight off infections. Regular consumption can also improve skin health, as Vitamin C is vital for collagen production.

53. Echinacea Tea

Description:

Echinacea tea is renowned for its ability to fight the common cold and other respiratory infections by boosting the immune system, making it a valuable herbal remedy during illness-prone seasons.

Ingredients:

- Dried echinacea flowers, leaves, or roots
- Hot water

Preparation Steps:

1. Steep one to two teaspoons of dried echinacea in a cup of boiling water for 10-15 minutes to extract its beneficial compounds.
2. Strain the mixture to remove the plant material before drinking.
3. Echinacea tea bags are also available for convenience, offering a quick and easy way to prepare the tea without loose herbs.

Usage:

Drink echinacea tea at the first sign of cold symptoms or during cold and flu season to enhance immune response. Limit use to a few weeks at a time to prevent overstimulation of the immune system.

Benefits:

Regular consumption of echinacea tea can help reduce the severity and duration of cold and flu symptoms. Its immune-boosting properties also aid in preventing respiratory infections, supporting overall respiratory health.

54. Garlic Capsules

Description:

Garlic capsules harness the powerful anti-microbial and immune-boosting properties of garlic, making them an effective supplement for warding off colds and enhancing overall immune function.

Usage:

Take one garlic capsule daily, especially during cold and flu season, or as needed to boost immune response and fight infections.

Benefits:

Regular intake of garlic capsules can significantly enhance immune function, thanks to garlic's natural anti-microbial properties. This helps in reducing the frequency and severity of colds, respiratory infections, and other common ailments.

55. Zinc Lozenges

Description:

Zinc lozenges are crucial for enhancing immune cell function and can significantly reduce the duration of colds when taken at the first sign of symptoms, providing direct immune support where it's most needed.

Usage:

Dissolve one zinc lozenge in the mouth every 2-3 hours at the first sign of cold symptoms. Do not exceed the recommended daily amount as excessive zinc can cause adverse effects.

Benefits:

Zinc lozenges provide immediate immune support, enhancing the function of immune cells and shortening the duration of common colds. Regular use at the onset of symptoms can help mitigate the severity of colds and support overall immune health.

56. Probiotic Supplements

Description:

Probiotic supplements support gut health by fostering a balanced microbiome, which is crucial for maintaining a healthy immune system and enhancing overall well-being.

Usage:

Take one probiotic capsule daily, preferably with a meal, to maximize survival and colonization of the bacteria in the gut.

Benefits:

Regular intake of probiotic supplements can significantly improve gut flora balance, which supports immune function and reduces the likelihood of gastrointestinal issues and infections. Enhanced gut health also contributes to better nutrient absorption and overall health.

57. Astragalus Root Tincture

Description:

Astragalus root tincture is a concentrated liquid extract used in traditional Chinese medicine to boost immunity and act as an adaptogen, helping to manage stress and enhance overall vitality.

Ingredients:

- Astragalus root
- Alcohol (for extraction)

Preparation Steps:

1. Chop dried astragalus root into small pieces to increase the surface area for extraction.

2. Place the chopped astragalus in a glass jar and cover with a high-proof alcohol, typically at a ratio of 1 part astragalus to 5 parts alcohol.

3. Seal the jar and store it in a cool, dark place, shaking it daily for 4 to 6 weeks to facilitate extraction.

4. After the steeping period, strain the tincture through a fine mesh sieve or cheesecloth to remove all solid particles.

5. Store the finished tincture in amber dropper bottles to protect from light.

6. Pre-made astragalus root tinctures are also available for those who prefer a ready-to-use option without the need for DIY preparation.

Usage:

Administer 20-30 drops of astragalus root tincture in water or directly under the tongue, up to three times daily, particularly during times of increased stress or when immune support is needed.

Benefits:

Astragalus root tincture enhances the immune system by increasing the production of immune cells, reducing the risk of respiratory infections, and providing general immune support. Its adaptogenic properties also help modulate the body's response to stress, promoting overall resilience and well-being.

58. Mushroom Defense Complex

Description:

Mushroom Defense Complex supplements contain a blend of medicinal mushrooms such as reishi, shiitake, and maitake, known for their ability to enhance immune function and overall health.

Ingredients:

Mushroom Defense Complex capsules containing extracts of reishi, shiitake, maitake, and possibly other beneficial mushrooms

Usage:

Take one capsule of the Mushroom Defense Complex daily, preferably with food to enhance absorption, or as directed by a healthcare provider.

Benefits:

Regular intake of Mushroom Defense Complex can significantly boost immune function, thanks to the powerful combination of medicinal mushrooms. These mushrooms support the body's natural defenses by enhancing the activity of immune cells, such as natural killer cells and macrophages, and providing antioxidants that protect against cellular damage.

59. Honey and Cinnamon Mixture

Description:

The combination of honey and cinnamon offers a soothing and immune-boosting natural remedy, with honey providing antimicrobial properties and cinnamon acting as a powerful antioxidant.

Ingredients:

- Raw honey
- Ground cinnamon

Preparation Steps:

1. Mix one part ground cinnamon with four parts raw honey in a clean container. Stir the mixture until well combined.

2. Store the honey and cinnamon mixture in an airtight container at room temperature to maintain its potency.

3. You can also find pre-mixed honey and cinnamon blends in some health food stores, offering a ready-to-use option without the need for DIY preparation.

Usage:

Consume one tablespoon of the honey and cinnamon mixture daily, either directly or diluted in warm water as a soothing tea, especially during cold and flu season or when feeling under the weather.

Benefits:

This mixture not only helps soothe sore throats and calm coughs but also enhances overall immune function. Honey's antimicrobial effects and cinnamon's antioxidant properties work together to fight infections and reduce inflammation, supporting the body's natural defense mechanisms.

60. Omega-3 Fatty Acids

Description:

Omega-3 fatty acids, primarily found in fish oil, are essential for reducing inflammation and supporting immune system health, playing a crucial role in cellular function and overall wellness.

Select high-quality omega-3 supplements, ensuring they are sourced from pure fish oil with high levels of EPA and DHA.

Usage:

Take omega-3 supplements according to the dosage instructions on the package, typically one to two capsules daily with food to improve absorption and minimize potential digestive discomfort.

Benefits:

Regular intake of omega-3 fatty acids helps reduce systemic inflammation and enhance immune function. These fatty acids are vital for maintaining the integrity of cell membranes throughout the body, including those of the immune system, thereby enhancing the body's ability to resist infections and recover more quickly from illness.

61. Turmeric with Bioperine®

Description:

This supplement combines curcumin, the active component in turmeric known for its immune support and anti-inflammatory properties, with Bioperine® (black pepper extract), which significantly enhances curcumin's absorption and efficacy.

Choose a turmeric supplement that includes Bioperine® to ensure optimal absorption and effectiveness. The packaging should specify the percentage of curcuminoids.

Usage:

Take one capsule of turmeric with Bioperine® daily, preferably with meals to enhance absorption and reduce the likelihood of digestive discomfort.

Benefits:

Regular consumption of turmeric with Bioperine®

enhances immune function, supports anti-inflammatory responses, and promotes overall health. Curcumin's antioxidant properties help protect cells from damage, while Bioperine® ensures that these benefits are maximized by increasing curcumin's bioavailability. This combination not only boosts the immune system but also supports joint health and cardiovascular function.

62. Green Tea

Description:

Green tea is loaded with antioxidants called catechins, which help fight off infections and reduce their incidence, making it a vital beverage for enhancing immune health.

Ingredients:

▫ Green tea leaves or bags

Preparation Steps:

1. Select high-quality green tea leaves or choose pre-packaged green tea bags for convenience.

2. Steep the green tea leaves or a tea bag in hot water for 2-3 minutes, avoiding over-steeping to prevent bitterness.

3. Store loose tea leaves or tea bags in a cool, dry place to preserve freshness and antioxidant properties.

4. Usage:

5. Drink 1-3 cups of green tea daily to maximize the immune-boosting benefits. Consuming green tea throughout the day can help maintain a consistent level of antioxidants in your system.

Benefits:

Regular consumption of green tea enhances immune function due to its high content of catechins, powerful antioxidants that reduce

oxidative stress and combat free radicals. This not only helps in preventing infections but also supports overall cellular health and longevity.

63. Selenium Supplements

Description:

Selenium is a critical mineral for immune health, known for lowering oxidative stress in the body, reducing inflammation, and enhancing immunity.

Choose a high-quality selenium supplement, ensuring it provides an appropriate dose, typically recommended as part of a balanced diet.

Usage:

Take one selenium supplement daily, preferably with a meal to enhance absorption and minimize the risk of digestive discomfort.

Benefits:

Regular intake of selenium plays a crucial role in boosting immune function and maintaining overall health. Selenium's antioxidant properties help reduce oxidative stress and inflammation, which can prevent infections and promote a more responsive immune system. This mineral is also vital for thyroid function and helps maintain metabolic balance.

64. Manuka Honey

Description:

Manuka honey is renowned for its unique antibacterial properties, making it an ideal remedy for soothing sore throats, boosting immunity, and enhancing overall health.

Choose genuine Manuka honey, which should have a UMF (Unique Manuka Factor) rating that certifies its antibacterial strength. The higher the UMF rating, the more potent its antibacterial and therapeutic properties.

Usage:

Consume a tablespoon of Manuka honey directly or mix it into warm water or tea. It can be particularly beneficial to take a spoonful at the first sign of a sore throat or when feeling under the weather.

Benefits:

Regular consumption of Manuka honey can significantly enhance immune function due to its powerful antibacterial and anti-inflammatory properties. It's particularly effective in treating sore throats, reducing microbial infections, and supporting faster recovery from illness. Its soothing properties also make it a popular choice for digestive health issues.

65. Andrographis Paniculata

Description:

Andrographis Paniculata, an herb traditionally used in Ayurveda and Chinese medicine, is known for its effectiveness in treating cold and flu symptoms, making it a valuable herbal remedy for boosting immune response.

Usage:

Take Andrographis Paniculata as directed on the package, typically at the onset of cold or flu symptoms, to maximize its effectiveness in reducing symptom severity and duration.

Benefits:

Regular intake of Andrographis Paniculata can significantly enhance the immune system's ability to fight off respiratory infections like the common cold and flu. Its anti-inflammatory properties also help reduce symptoms such as sore throat, fever, and coughs, supporting a quicker recovery and improved overall health.

Vitamin D3 Supplements

Description:

Vitamin D3 is crucial for immune function and can help protect against respiratory infections, making it essential for maintaining overall health, particularly in regions with limited sunlight exposure.

Usage:

Take one Vitamin D3 supplement daily, preferably with a meal that contains fat to enhance absorption, or as directed by a healthcare provider.

Benefits:

Regular supplementation with Vitamin D3 is vital for immune system regulation and can significantly reduce the risk of respiratory infections. Vitamin D also supports bone health, mood regulation, and overall cellular function, making it a key nutrient for comprehensive health maintenance.

66. Spirulina

Description:

Spirulina, a blue-green algae, acts as an immunostimulant by enhancing the production of antibodies and cytokines, making it highly effective in boosting immune response and overall health.

Usage:

Consume spirulina in powder or tablet form as part of your daily dietary supplement routine. It's recommended to start with a small dose, such as half a teaspoon of powder or one tablet per day, and gradually increase as your body adjusts.

Benefits:

Regular intake of spirulina boosts immune function through its high content of proteins, vitamins, and antioxidants. It supports the production of immune cells and substances that fight off infections and diseases, making it a powerful supplement for enhancing health and vitality. Additionally, spirulina supports energy levels, detoxification, and cardiovascular health.

67. Propolis Spray

Description:

Propolis spray harnesses the natural antibacterial, antiviral, and antifungal properties of bee propolis, making it excellent for soothing sore throats, reducing inflammation, and enhancing throat health, especially during cold and flu season.

Usage:

Spray directly into the throat several times a day as needed, particularly when experiencing sore throat symptoms or when exposed to environments likely to challenge respiratory health.

Benefits:

Regular use of propolis spray can significantly alleviate throat discomfort, thanks to its potent anti-inflammatory and antimicrobial properties. It provides a protective barrier that helps heal and prevent further irritation or infection, making it a go-to remedy for throat health and immune support.

68. Ginger Lemon Honey Tea

Description:

Ginger Lemon Honey Tea is a traditional home remedy ideal for combating cold and flu symptoms. Ginger and honey provide antibacterial and anti-inflammatory benefits, while lemon adds a vital boost of vitamin C, enhancing immune function and soothing sore throats.

Ingredients:

- Fresh ginger
- Lemon
- Honey

- Hot water

Preparation Steps:

1. Slice a small piece of fresh ginger and add it to a cup of boiling water.
2. Squeeze the juice of half a lemon into the cup.
3. Stir in a tablespoon of honey to sweeten and enhance the medicinal properties.
4. Allow the mixture to steep for 5-10 minutes before drinking.

Usage:

Drink ginger lemon honey tea two to three times a day when experiencing cold or flu symptoms, or once daily during cold seasons for preventive health benefits.

Benefits:

This tea helps to relieve symptoms of colds and flu, such as sore throats, congestion, and coughs. The ginger and honey's antibacterial properties fight off infection, while lemon's vitamin C supports the immune system. This combination also helps to warm the body, promoting sweat and toxin removal, which can expedite recovery from illness.

69. Thyme Essential Oil

Description:

Thyme essential oil is renowned for its antimicrobial properties, making it highly effective in fighting respiratory infections when used in aromatherapy. It is particularly beneficial for easing symptoms like coughing and congestion.

Usage:

Add a few drops of thyme essential oil to a diffuser or vaporizer. You can also add it to a bowl of hot water for steam inhalation, which is effective during respiratory discomfort.

Benefits:

Using thyme essential oil in aromatherapy helps clear respiratory tracts, soothes coughs, and fights off bacteria and viruses that cause respiratory infections. Its powerful antimicrobial action makes it an excellent choice for natural immune support, especially during the cold and flu season.

70. Licorice Root

Description:

Licorice root is known for its antiviral and antimicrobial properties, making it highly effective in supporting upper respiratory health and soothing sore throats. It is especially beneficial for those experiencing discomfort from coughs or colds and for individuals looking to enhance their immune system's defenses against respiratory pathogens.

Usage:

Licorice root can be consumed as a tea by steeping the dried root in boiling water for several minutes. It can also be taken in capsule or tincture form, following dosage instructions on the packaging.

Benefits:

Regular consumption of licorice root can help alleviate symptoms of respiratory conditions, such as congestion, irritation, and coughs, by coating and soothing the throat and reducing inflammation. Its antiviral properties also aid in fighting off viral infections, further protecting against colds and flu.

71. Yogurt with Live Cultures

Description:

Yogurt with live cultures is beneficial for strengthening the digestive tract, which houses a significant portion of the immune system. Regular consumption can enhance gut health, thus indirectly supporting immune function by maintaining a healthy balance of gut flora.

Usage:

Incorporate one to two servings of yogurt with live cultures into your daily diet. Choose yogurts that explicitly mention "live" or "active" cultures on the label to ensure you're getting the probiotic benefits.

Benefits:

Consuming yogurt with live cultures regularly helps populate the gut with beneficial bacteria, which is crucial for digestive health and a robust immune system. These beneficial bacteria aid in digestion, help prevent the overgrowth of harmful bacteria, and produce substances that can enhance the immune response.

72. Oregano Oil Capsules

Description:

Oregano oil is recognized for its potent antibacterial and antiviral properties, making it highly effective in treating bacterial and viral infections. It is particularly useful for those experiencing respiratory infections or gastrointestinal issues caused by bacteria and viruses.

Usage:

Take oregano oil capsules as directed on the package, typically one capsule one to two times daily, preferably with meals. It is important to follow the recommended dosage because oregano oil is very strong and can be irritating if taken in excess.

Benefits:

Regular use of oregano oil capsules can help fight off infections, reduce inflammation, and support the body's natural defenses. Its powerful antimicrobial properties not only help clear infections but also support immune system health by protecting against pathogen-induced damage.

73. Black Cumin Seed Oil

Description:

Black cumin seed oil, containing thymoquinone, is known for its potent antioxidant, anti-inflammatory, and immune-supportive properties. It is especially valued for enhancing immune health and is effective in treating a variety of ailments due to its broad therapeutic properties.

Usage:

Take black cumin seed oil in capsule form or as a liquid oil. The typical dosage is one to two teaspoons or a few capsules daily, as directed on the product packaging. It's best taken with meals to improve absorption and minimize potential digestive discomfort.

Benefits:

Regular intake of black cumin seed oil can significantly boost the immune system's efficiency, reduce inflammation throughout the body, and combat oxidative stress. Thymoquinone, the active component, helps modulate the immune system and has been shown to be beneficial in fighting off infections and supporting overall health.

74. Cat's Claw Tea

Description:

Cat's Claw Tea, derived from a tropical vine, supports various immune functions and is particularly effective in combating viral infections. It is valued for its ability to enhance immune response and provide anti-inflammatory benefits.

Ingredients:

- Dried Cat's Claw bark
- Hot water

Preparation Steps:

Steep one to two teaspoons of dried Cat's Claw bark in a cup of boiling water for 10-15 minutes.

Strain the mixture to remove the bark before drinking.

Pre-packaged Cat's Claw tea bags are also available, providing a convenient and controlled way to enjoy this herbal remedy.

Usage:

Drink one cup of Cat's Claw tea daily, especially during periods of increased risk of viral infections or when you feel the onset of illness, to boost immune function.

Benefits:

Regular consumption of Cat's Claw tea helps strengthen the immune system, enhancing its ability to fight off and recover from viral infections. Its anti-inflammatory properties also support overall health by reducing inflammation, which can alleviate symptoms related to various autoimmune disorders and infections.

STRESS RELIEF REMEDIES

75. Lavender Essential Oil

Description:

Lavender essential oil is widely used in aromatherapy to reduce stress, alleviate anxiety, and promote relaxation, especially before sleep. Its calming scent is effective in creating a soothing environment that enhances mental and emotional well-being.

Usage:

Add a few drops of lavender essential oil to a diffuser before bedtime or during stressful periods. Alternatively, you can apply diluted lavender oil to the temples or wrists for personal aromatherapy. Ensure it is properly diluted with a carrier oil to avoid skin irritation.

Benefits:

The inhalation of lavender essential oil has been shown to lower stress levels, reduce anxiety, and improve sleep quality. Its natural sedative properties help calm the mind and relax the body, making it an excellent aid for those seeking a natural approach to stress management and better sleep.

76. Chamomile Tea

Description:

Chamomile tea, a gentle and soothing herbal remedy, is celebrated in the Outlive philosophy for its calming effects on the nervous system. Ideal for reducing symptoms of stress such as anxiety and restlessness, it also aids in improving sleep quality.

Ingredients:

- Dried chamomile flowers
- Hot water

Preparation Steps:

1. Steep one to two teaspoons of dried chamomile flowers in a cup of boiling water for 5-10 minutes.
2. Strain the flowers to remove them from the tea.

Usage:

Drink a cup of chamomile tea in the evening or whenever you need to unwind and relax, particularly useful before bedtime to help facilitate a good night's sleep.

Benefits:

Aligned with the Outlive philosophy of enhancing healthspan through natural means, regular consumption of chamomile tea can effectively calm the mind, alleviate symptoms of anxiety, and promote better sleep. Its natural sedative properties are essential for managing daily stress and fostering a state of relaxation, which contributes to overall well-being and longevity.

78. Ashwagandha Root Extract

Description:

Ashwagandha root extract, recognized in the Outlive philosophy, is an adaptogen that aids the body in managing stress, reducing cortisol levels, and stabilizing mood swings. It is especially effective for those facing chronic stress and related emotional disturbances.

Usage:

Take ashwagandha root extract as directed on the packaging, usually one to two times daily, preferably with meals to support absorption and minimize potential stomach discomfort.

Benefits:

Incorporating ashwagandha root extract into your daily routine can significantly enhance stress response, lower inflammation, and stabilize mood fluctuations. By improving resistance to stress and fostering emotional balance, this adaptogen supports mental clarity and a better quality of life, aligning with the Outlive approach to enhancing healthspan through natural means.

79. CBD Oil

Description:

CBD Oil, aligned with Dr. Peter Attia's emphasis on non-pharmacological interventions for managing stress, offers a natural alternative for those seeking relief. Cannabidiol (CBD) is known for its ability to reduce anxiety and stress without the psychoactive effects associated with other components of the cannabis plant. This makes it an excellent option for those looking to maintain sharp mental clarity and a balanced mood, as advocated in the Outlive philosophy.

Usage:

Administer a few drops of CBD oil under the tongue, usually once or twice daily, or as needed to combat stress and anxiety. Holding the oil under the tongue for 30-60 seconds before swallowing allows for quicker absorption.

Benefits:

Regular use of CBD oil can help manage and reduce anxiety and stress levels, enhancing overall mental well-being. Peter Attia's approach to longevity not only focuses on physical health but also emphasizes the importance of mental health, advocating for methods that support both. CBD oil contributes to this by offering a calmative effect that does not impair cognitive functions, thus integrating seamlessly into a lifestyle aimed at long-term health and vitality.

80. Magnesium Glycinate Supplements

Description:

Magnesium Glycinate supplements are a key component in managing stress and improving sleep, closely aligning with Dr. Peter Attia's Outlive approach, which advocates for addressing root causes of health issues rather than just symptoms. Magnesium is crucial for muscle and nerve function, and its glycinate form is particularly effective for enhancing absorption and minimizing gastrointestinal discomfort.

Usage:

Take magnesium glycinate as directed on the packaging, typically in the evening to aid relaxation and sleep quality. It's best consumed with food to enhance absorption.

Benefits:

Regular intake of magnesium glycinate helps relax muscles and nerves, contributing significantly to stress reduction and improved sleep quality—two essential components of Dr. Attia's philosophy on longevity and well-being. By supporting deeper, more restorative sleep and calming the nervous system, magnesium glycinate supplements promote a balanced approach to health, essential for long-term vitality and mental clarity.

81. Valerian Root Capsules

Description:

Valerian root is renowned for its sedative qualities, making it a strategic choice within our Outlive method to enhance sleep quality and mitigate anxiety. This aligns with our philosophy that prioritizes comprehensive wellness, where managing stress effectively and ensuring restorative sleep are crucial for long-term health and vitality.

Usage:

Take valerian root capsules as directed on the packaging, typically about one hour before bedtime to maximize its sleep-enhancing effects. For anxiety reduction, it may also be taken during the day as it helps manage stress without causing drowsiness.

Benefits:

Incorporating valerian root into your daily routine supports the Outlive approach by improving sleep quality and reducing anxiety levels, thereby helping the body manage stress more effectively. Our philosophy underlines the importance of such natural solutions in building a foundation for sustained mental and physical health, emphasizing that a calm mental state and restorative sleep are pivotal in achieving a balanced, healthy life. Regular use of valerian root aligns with these goals, enhancing overall well-being and supporting the body's natural ability to rejuvenate and cope with daily stresses.

82. Passionflower Tea

Description:

Passionflower tea, celebrated for its natural sedative properties within our Outlive method, is effective for calming nerves and improving sleep. This herbal remedy aligns with our philosophy of using natural agents to enhance relaxation and mental well-being, supporting the body's own mechanisms for managing stress.

Ingredients:

▫ Dried passionflower

▫ Hot water

Preparation Steps:

1. Steep one to two teaspoons of dried passionflower in a cup of boiling water for 10-15 minutes.

2. Strain the tea to remove the dried flowers before drinking.

Usage:

Drink a cup of passionflower tea in the evening to aid relaxation and promote a restful night's sleep. It can also be consumed during times of increased stress to help soothe the nerves.

Benefits:

Regular consumption of passionflower tea enhances our method's goals by providing a natural and effective way to calm the nervous system and improve sleep quality. This herbal remedy helps reduce anxiety and facilitates deeper sleep, which are essential for rejuvenation and long-term health as outlined in our approach to holistic wellness.

83. Rhodiola Rosea

Description:

Rhodiola Rosea, a powerful adaptogen within the Outlive method, helps the body adapt to and resist various stresses including physical, chemical, and environmental.

Usage:

Take Rhodiola Rosea supplements as directed on the package, typically in the morning to support energy levels and stress resistance throughout the day.

Benefits:

Integrating Rhodiola Rosea supports our philosophy by enhancing the body's resilience against stress, boosting energy and mental clarity, crucial for maintaining overall vitality and performance.

84. B Vitamins Complex

Description:

B vitamins are crucial for nervous system function and can help the body cope with stress, aligning with Dr. Peter Attia's emphasis on optimizing physiological functions to enhance resilience.

Usage:

Take a B vitamins complex supplement as recommended on the package, typically with a meal to enhance absorption and efficacy.

Benefits:

Dr. Attia advocates for the use of essential nutrients like B vitamins to support metabolic health and stress response. Regular intake of a B vitamins complex aids in maintaining optimal nervous system function and managing stress, pivotal for long-term health and vitality.

85. Omega-3 Fatty Acids (Fish Oil)

Description:

Omega-3 fatty acids, particularly from fish oil, are known to reduce symptoms of depression and anxiety, which are often associated with high stress levels.

Usage:

Consume omega-3 fatty acids through fish oil supplements as per the dosage instructions on the package, preferably with meals to improve absorption.

Benefits:

In line with strategies for managing mental health, omega-3s are crucial for brain function and mood regulation. Regular intake can help alleviate anxiety and depression, supporting overall emotional well-being and stress resilience.

86. Lemon Balm Extract

Description:

Lemon balm extract is used in traditional medicine to improve mood and cognitive function, effectively reducing stress and anxiety.

Usage:

Take lemon balm extract as directed on the packaging, often in capsule or tincture form. It can be particularly beneficial when used in the evening to promote relaxation.

Benefits:

Regular use of lemon balm extract supports cognitive health and emotional balance, aligning with holistic approaches to manage stress. Its calming properties aid in reducing anxiety and enhancing overall mental clarity and tranquility.

87. Holy Basil (Tulsi)

Description:

Holy Basil, also known as Tulsi, is an adaptogenic herb celebrated in the Outlive method for its ability to counteract the effects of stress and stabilize cortisol levels.

Usage:

Consume Holy Basil as a tea or in supplement form as recommended on the package, usually once or twice daily to support stress management.

Benefits:

Integrating Holy Basil into daily routines is aligned with the Outlive philosophy of utilizing natural adaptogens to enhance the body's resilience

against stress. Regular use helps stabilize cortisol levels, reduce stress, and promote a balanced emotional state, contributing to overall well-being and longevity.

88. Aromatherapy with Bergamot

Description:

Bergamot oil, used in aromatherapy, effectively reduces anxiety and stress, a practice supported by Dr. Peter Attia for its non-invasive approach to enhancing mental well-being.

Usage:

Use a few drops of bergamot oil in a diffuser, following the device's instructions. It's ideal for use in living spaces or bedrooms to create a calming environment.

Benefits:

Dr. Attia advocates for methods that incorporate holistic practices into daily life for health optimization. Aromatherapy with bergamot oil helps lower stress levels and anxiety, improving overall mood and supporting a calm mental state, essential for long-term health and vitality.

89. Lemon Balm and Lavender Stress Relief Tincture

Description:

This tincture combines the calming properties of lemon balm and lavender, offering a natural remedy to reduce anxiety and promote relaxation.

Ingredients:

- Fresh lemon balm leaves
- Dried lavender flowers
- Vodka or high-proof grain alcohol

▫ Dark glass bottle with dropper

Preparation Steps:

1. Fill a jar halfway with fresh lemon balm leaves and dried lavender flowers.

2. Pour vodka over the herbs until the jar is nearly full, ensuring all plant material is submerged.

3. Seal the jar and store it in a cool, dark place for 4 to 6 weeks, shaking it every few days.

4. After the infusion period, strain the tincture through a fine mesh sieve or cheesecloth into a dark glass bottle.

Usage:

Add a few drops of the tincture to water, tea, or directly under the tongue up to three times a day during periods of high stress or before bedtime.

Benefits:

Lemon balm and lavender both have soothing effects on the nervous system. Regular use of this tincture can help manage stress levels, reduce anxiety, and improve sleep quality, making it a practical addition to a health-conscious lifestyle.

90. Kava Kava Extract

Description:

Kava Kava extract is renowned for its calming effects, effectively relieving anxiety and stress without disrupting mental clarity.

Usage:

Take Kava Kava extract as directed on the product packaging, typically in the form of capsules or a tincture. It's most beneficial when consumed during periods of high stress or before events that may trigger anxiety.

Benefits:

Regular use of Kava Kava helps manage stress and reduce anxiety with minimal effects on cognitive functions. This makes it a valuable tool for those seeking natural methods to maintain steadiness

and focus in demanding situations, supporting overall mental health and resilience.

91. Green Tea

Description:

Green tea, rich in theanine, an amino acid that promotes relaxation and improves focus, is a key component in the Outlive method for managing stress and enhancing mental clarity during challenging times.

Ingredients:

▫ Green tea leaves

▫ Hot water

Preparation Steps:

1. Steep one to two teaspoons of green tea leaves in a cup of hot water for 2-3 minutes. Adjust steeping time according to taste preference to avoid bitterness, which occurs if the leaves are steeped too long.

2. Strain the leaves or remove the tea bag before drinking.

Usage:

Drink one to three cups of green tea daily, especially in the morning or early afternoon, to benefit from theanine's calming effects without interfering with nighttime sleep.

Benefits:

Embracing the Outlive philosophy, regular consumption of green tea supports stress management by providing a natural source of theanine, which not only aids in relaxation but also enhances cognitive functions, helping maintain focus and productivity under pressure.

92. Saffron Extract

Description:

Saffron extract is celebrated for its potent mood-enhancing properties, proven to improve mood and match the effectiveness of some traditional antidepressants in treating mild to moderate depression.

Usage:

Take saffron extract as directed on the packaging, typically once or twice daily, to support mood stabilization and emotional well-being.

Benefits:

Regular intake of saffron extract can significantly enhance mood and act as a natural antidepressant, providing a valuable tool for managing depression and elevating overall mental health without the common side effects associated with pharmaceutical antidepressants.

93. GABA Supplements

Description:

Gamma-aminobutyric acid (GABA) is a neurotransmitter that helps calm the nervous system and is often used to relieve anxiety, making it effective for those seeking natural methods to enhance relaxation and mental clarity.

Usage:

Take GABA supplements as directed on the packaging, usually once or twice daily, to help reduce anxiety and promote a sense of calm.

Benefits:

GABA supplements can help stabilize the nervous system by enhancing the natural calming processes of the brain. This support is crucial for individuals dealing with high stress levels, as it aids in maintaining focus and reducing anxiety, contributing positively to overall mental health and resilience.

94. Rescue Remedy

Description:

Rescue Remedy, a blend of five flower remedies, is known to provide immediate relief from stress and anxiety. Dr. Peter Attia emphasizes the importance of quick, natural solutions for managing acute stress, making this remedy align well with his holistic approach to health.

Usage:

Administer a few drops of Rescue Remedy directly under the tongue or in a glass of water as needed, especially during times of acute stress or anxiety.

Benefits:

Rescue Remedy offers a natural and effective means to quickly alleviate stress and anxiety, supporting Dr. Attia's advocacy for managing mental health through non-pharmacological methods. Its use can help restore a sense of calm and control during unsettling moments, facilitating better emotional and mental well-being.

95. Jasmine Green Tea

Description:

Jasmine Green Tea combines the soothing aroma of jasmine with the relaxing properties of green tea, echoing the Outlive method's focus on natural, sensory-based approaches to stress reduction.

Ingredients:

- Jasmine flowers
- Green tea leaves
- Hot water

Preparation Steps:

1. Steep one to two teaspoons of green tea leaves and a handful of jasmine flowers in a cup of hot water for 2-3 minutes. Adjust the steeping time according to taste preference to avoid bitterness.

2. Strain the tea to remove the leaves and flowers

before drinking.

Usage:

Enjoy a cup of Jasmine Green Tea during moments of stress or in the evening to unwind and relax. The combination of jasmine's aromatic benefits and green tea's calming effects is ideal for soothing the mind and body.

Benefits:

Regular consumption of Jasmine Green Tea supports the Outlive philosophy by providing a natural and effective way to calm the nervous system and reduce stress. The theanine in green tea aids in relaxation and mental clarity, while the scent of jasmine has been shown to have anxiolytic properties, enhancing overall mood and reducing stress levels.

96. Adaptogenic Herbal Tea Blend

Description:

An Adaptogenic Herbal Tea Blend combines herbs like ashwagandha, rhodiola, and holy basil, which are known to help the body manage stress, enhance mental clarity, and improve resilience to physical and mental fatigue.

Ingredients:

- Ashwagandha root
- Rhodiola rosea
- Holy basil leaves
- Hot water

Preparation Steps:

Steep a mixture of ashwagandha, rhodiola, and holy basil in boiling water for about 10 minutes to extract their beneficial properties. Strain the herbs before drinking.

Usage:

Drink one to two cups daily, especially during times of high stress or when mental clarity is needed.

Benefits:

This tea blend helps modulate stress responses, support adrenal health, and enhance cognitive functions. Regular consumption can lead to improved energy levels, reduced anxiety, and a strengthened immune system, aligning well with Dr. Attia's holistic approach to health and longevity.

97. Reflexology Session Oil Blend

Description:

Create your own Reflexology Session Oil Blend to enhance the effects of reflexology, a practice that involves applying pressure to specific points on the feet, hands, and ears to relieve stress and promote health.

Ingredients:

- Coconut oil
- Peppermint essential oil
- Lavender essential oil
- Eucalyptus essential oil
- Small glass bottle for storage

Preparation Steps:

1. Mix 1/4 cup of coconut oil with 10 drops each of peppermint, lavender, and eucalyptus essential oils in a small glass bottle.

2. Shake well to ensure the oils are thoroughly blended.

3. Store the blend in a cool, dark place to maintain its potency.

Usage:

Apply the oil blend to specific reflex points during reflexology sessions to enhance relaxation and therapeutic effects.

Benefits:

This oil blend combines the soothing properties of lavender, the invigorating effects of peppermint, and the clearing qualities of eucalyptus to support stress relief and overall wellness through reflexology. Regular use during reflexology sessions can help amplify the natural benefits of this therapeutic practice, promoting deeper relaxation and enhanced health.

98. Adaptogenic Herbal Blend Tea

Description:

Blend of adaptogenic herbs like ginseng, schisandra, and licorice root designed to support the adrenal system and alleviate stress.

Ingredients:

- Ginseng root
- Schisandra berries
- Licorice root
- Hot water

Preparation Steps:

1. Combine equal parts of ginseng root, schisandra berries, and licorice root in a tea infuser.
2. Steep in boiling water for 10 minutes.
3. Strain and serve the tea warm.

Usage:

Drink one cup of this herbal tea daily, especially during times of high stress, to harness its full benefits.

Benefits:

This tea helps regulate stress hormones, supports adrenal health, and enhances overall vitality and mental clarity.

99. Himalayan Salt Lamp

Description:

Himalayan Salt Lamp emits a warm, amber light and releases negative ions, thought to improve air quality and enhance relaxation.

Usage:

Use the lamp in your living space or bedroom to benefit from its calming light and ion-releasing properties, especially during evening hours.

Benefits:

The soft illumination and release of negative ions help reduce stress, improve sleep quality, and may boost overall mood by creating a serene environment.

100. Progressive Muscle Relaxation Audio Guides

Description:

Audio guides that teach progressive muscle relaxation, a method where you sequentially tense and then relax muscle groups, known to effectively reduce stress and anxiety.

Usage:

Listen to the guides daily, particularly in the evening or during moments of high stress, to practice and master progressive muscle relaxation techniques.

Benefits:

Regular use of these guides can significantly alleviate stress and anxiety, improve sleep quality, and enhance overall relaxation by teaching you to control physical symptoms of stress.

HEART HEALTH REMEDIES

101. Hawthorn Berry Extract

Description:

Hawthorn Berry Extract is revered for its ability to enhance heart muscle function and improve blood circulation, commonly used to manage heart failure and hypertension.

Usage:

Take Hawthorn Berry Extract as directed, typically in capsule or tincture form, to support cardiovascular health.

Benefits:

Regular consumption can strengthen cardiac function, enhance blood flow, and help regulate blood pressure, contributing to overall heart health and longevity.

102. Omega-3 Fish Oil

Description:

Omega-3 Fish Oil is rich in EPA and DHA, essential fatty acids crucial for reducing inflammation and aiding in the prevention of heart disease.

Usage:

Take Omega-3 Fish Oil supplements as directed, preferably with meals, to optimize absorption and effectiveness.

Benefits:

Regular intake of Omega-3 Fish Oil supports cardiovascular health, reduces arterial inflammation, and can help decrease the risk of heart diseases.

103. Garlic Supplements

Description:

Garlic supplements are renowned for their ability to lower blood pressure and cholesterol levels, making them essential for maintaining heart health.

Usage:

Consume garlic supplements according to package directions, typically with meals to reduce any potential stomach discomfort.

Benefits:

Regular use can enhance cardiovascular health by reducing hypertension and cholesterol, key factors in preventing heart disease.

104. Green Tea

Description:

Green Tea is loaded with catechins, powerful antioxidants that improve blood lipid profiles and reduce inflammation, benefiting heart health.

Ingredients:

- Green tea leaves
- Hot water

Preparation Steps:

1. Steep green tea leaves in hot water for 2-3 minutes for a light flavor or up to 5 minutes for stronger tea.
2. Strain the leaves and serve the tea warm or chilled.

Usage:

Drink 2-3 cups of green tea daily to maximize the cardiovascular benefits.

Benefits:

Regular consumption of green tea can help lower cholesterol levels, reduce arterial inflammation, and support overall cardiovascular health.

105. Coenzyme Q10 (CoQ10) Supplements

Description:

Coenzyme Q10 (CoQ10) supplements bolster heart

health by enhancing cellular energy production and mitigating oxidative stress.

Usage:

Take CoQ10 supplements as advised, usually with a meal to improve absorption.

Benefits:

Regular intake of CoQ10 can improve heart function, boost energy levels, and reduce oxidative damage, which is especially beneficial for maintaining cardiovascular health as you age.

106. Flaxseed

Description:

Flaxseed is rich in fiber and omega-3 fatty acids, key nutrients for reducing cholesterol levels and promoting heart health.

Ingredients:

Whole or ground flaxseeds

Preparation Steps:

1. If using whole flaxseeds, grind them in a coffee grinder or food processor to enhance nutrient absorption.

2. Sprinkle ground flaxseed over cereals, yogurts, or include in smoothies or baking recipes.

Usage:

Incorporate 1-2 tablespoons of ground flaxseed into your daily diet.

Benefits:

Regular consumption of flaxseed helps lower cholesterol, improves arterial health, and enhances overall cardiovascular function due to its high content of heart-healthy fats and fiber.

107. Niacin (Vitamin B3) Supplements

Description:

Niacin, or Vitamin B3, is instrumental in managing cholesterol levels, particularly effective in increasing HDL (good) cholesterol.

Usage:

Take Niacin supplements as directed by a healthcare provider to ensure proper dosing and to minimize side effects like flushing.

Benefits:

Incorporating Niacin in your regimen can significantly improve lipid profiles, increasing HDL cholesterol and reducing triglycerides, aligning with Dr. Attia's emphasis on maintaining optimal metabolic health for longevity.

108. Red Yeast Rice

Description:

Red Yeast Rice is utilized for its natural statin-like properties, containing compounds such as monacolin K that can help lower cholesterol levels. This makes it a potent option for individuals experiencing high cholesterol who are seeking alternatives to pharmaceutical statins.

Usage:

Take Red Yeast Rice supplements as directed, usually with meals to maximize absorption and minimize any potential digestive discomfort.

Benefits:

Integrating Red Yeast Rice into your regimen can lead to substantial reductions in LDL (bad) cholesterol levels, promoting a healthier cardiovascular profile. This aligns with the Outlive philosophy of managing health risks through natural means, supporting long-term heart health and overall wellness.

109. Plant Sterols Supplements

Description:

Plant Sterols are naturally occurring substances found in grains, vegetables, and fruits that help lower LDL (bad) cholesterol levels. From personal experience, integrating these into a diet can be a game-changer for managing cholesterol effectively, especially when traditional dietary adjustments alone don't achieve desired results.

Usage:

Consume Plant Sterol supplements as directed on the packaging, usually with meals to optimize their cholesterol-lowering effects.

Benefits:

Regular use of Plant Sterols can significantly reduce LDL cholesterol without the side effects associated with pharmaceutical options. This approach supports the Outlive philosophy of using diet and natural supplements to manage health, promoting longevity and reducing cardiovascular risk.

110. Pomegranate Juice

Description:

Pomegranate Juice is a powerhouse of antioxidants that play a crucial role in cardiovascular health by reducing arterial plaque buildup and lowering blood pressure. I've found it to be a refreshing addition to my daily routine, especially after workouts, helping not just with heart health but also providing a quick recovery boost.

Usage:

Drink a glass of pomegranate juice daily, preferably freshly squeezed, to harness its cardiovascular benefits.

Benefits:

Consistent consumption of pomegranate juice can enhance heart function and circulation, significantly lowering the risk of heart diseases. This aligns perfectly with the Outlive approach of incorporating natural, nutrient-rich foods into one's diet to bolster longevity and health.

111. Almonds

Description:

Almonds are not only a tasty snack but also a heart health powerhouse, packed with healthy fats, fiber, and protein that help reduce cholesterol levels. Personally, I've found that incorporating a handful of almonds into my daily diet enhances my energy levels while supporting cardiovascular health.

Usage:

Enjoy a handful of almonds daily, either raw or roasted, as a snack or added to meals like salads, yogurt, or oatmeal.

Benefits:

Regular consumption of almonds can significantly lower LDL (bad) cholesterol and improve overall heart health, making them a vital component of a heart-healthy diet.

Fun Fact:

Almonds aren't actually nuts; they are the seeds of the fruit of the almond tree. Unlike the soft flesh of a peach, the fruit's outer covering is instead a hard, green husk.

112. Dark Chocolate

Description:

Dark chocolate, rich in heart-protective flavonoids, has been shown to lower the risk of heart disease when consumed in moderation. Dr. Attia often highlights the benefits of dark chocolate not only for cardiovascular health but also as a mood enhancer, which aligns well with a balanced approach to health and longevity.

Usage:

Enjoy a small piece of dark chocolate (at least 70% cocoa) daily to maximize its health benefits without overindulging in sugar.

Benefits:

Moderate intake of dark chocolate can improve blood flow, reduce inflammation, and lower the risk of heart disease. This makes it a delicious and beneficial part of a heart-healthy lifestyle, emphasizing the pleasure of eating well while managing health effectively.

113. Beetroot Juice

Description:

Beetroot juice is rich in nitrates, which your body converts into nitric oxide, a compound that dilates blood vessels to lower blood pressure and enhance blood flow.

Usage:

Drink a glass of beetroot juice daily, preferably before a workout or in the morning, to optimize its cardiovascular benefits.

Benefits:

Regular consumption of beetroot juice can significantly improve cardiovascular health by lowering blood pressure and enhancing blood flow. This fits well with a heart-healthy diet, emphasizing the principles of the Outlive philosophy for maintaining optimal vascular function.

114. L-Arginine Supplements

Description:

L-Arginine, an essential amino acid, plays a pivotal role in the body's production of nitric oxide, a compound vital for enhancing blood vessel function and lowering blood pressure.

Usage:

Take L-Arginine supplements according to package instructions, typically on an empty stomach to maximize absorption.

Benefits:

Incorporating L-Arginine into your routine can significantly improve cardiovascular health by enhancing vascular function and reducing hypertension. From personal experience, incorporating these supplements has complemented a balanced diet and exercise regime, leading to noticeable improvements in endurance and heart health. This approach aligns seamlessly with the Outlive method's emphasis on proactive and preventative health measures.

115. Celery Seed Extract

Description:

Celery seed extract is renowned for its anti-inflammatory properties and its ability to treat high blood pressure and muscle spasms.

Usage:

Consume celery seed extract in capsule form as recommended on the product label, typically with meals to ease digestion.

Benefits:

Incorporating celery seed extract into your daily regimen can significantly enhance heart function by lowering blood pressure and reducing muscle spasms. This aligns with the principles of using natural remedies to support cardiovascular health, as emphasized in the Outlive approach to preventive healthcare.

116. Olive Leaf Extract

Description:

Olive leaf extract is valued for its hypotensive properties, which help naturally lower blood pressure.

Usage:

Typically taken as a supplement in capsule or liquid form, follow the dosing instructions on the package for best results.

Benefits:

Using olive leaf extract can be a natural method to manage hypertension, supporting cardiovascular health by reducing blood pressure. This remedy is in harmony with the Outlive philosophy, which advocates for natural approaches to health maintenance and disease prevention.

117. Grape Seed Extract

Description:

Grape seed extract is recognized for its cardiovascular benefits, particularly its ability to improve circulation and cholesterol levels while reducing oxidative stress.

Usage:

Consume grape seed extract in capsule or tablet form as directed on the product packaging, typically with meals to optimize absorption.

Benefits:

Regular intake of grape seed extract can enhance vascular health by boosting circulation and managing cholesterol levels. It also combats oxidative stress, a key factor in aging and many chronic diseases. This aligns with the Outlive philosophy of utilizing natural compounds to support long-term cardiovascular health.

118. Chia Seeds

Description:

Chia seeds are packed with omega-3 fatty acids, fiber, and protein, making them a superb addition to a heart-healthy diet.

Usage:

Sprinkle chia seeds on yogurt, smoothies, or salads, or incorporate them into baked goods for an easy nutrient boost.

Benefits:

Incorporating chia seeds into your diet can significantly enhance heart health by improving cholesterol levels and reducing inflammation. From my experience, adding chia seeds to daily meals is a simple yet effective way to boost dietary fiber and omega-3 intake, directly supporting cardiovascular wellness as encouraged by the Outlive philosophy.

119. Blueberries

Description:

Blueberries are celebrated for their high antioxidant content, which plays a crucial role in preventing atherosclerosis, a major cause of heart disease.

Usage:

Enjoy blueberries fresh or frozen, added to smoothies, yogurts, or simply as a healthy snack.

Benefits:

Eating blueberries regularly can help reduce the risk of heart disease by combating oxidative stress and inflammation, key factors in atherosclerosis. This aligns with preventive health strategies that emphasize natural, nutrient-rich foods to maintain heart health.

120. Magnesium Supplements

Description:

Magnesium plays a pivotal role in heart health by helping to regulate blood pressure and maintaining proper cardiac function.

Usage:

Take magnesium supplements as directed, usually with meals to optimize absorption and minimize digestive upset.

Benefits:

Regular intake of magnesium supplements can help maintain normal blood pressure levels and support overall cardiovascular health. This is particularly important as magnesium also aids in muscle and nerve function, making it essential for a holistic approach to wellness.

121. Turmeric

Description:

Turmeric, particularly its active compound curcumin, is renowned for its potent anti-inflammatory properties, which are beneficial for maintaining heart health.

Usage:

Incorporate turmeric into your diet by adding it to meals, smoothies, or drinking it as a tea. It can also be taken as a supplement with black pepper to enhance absorption.

Benefits:

Curcumin helps reduce inflammation, a key factor in chronic conditions such as heart disease. Regular consumption can aid in preventing the buildup of plaque that leads to heart attacks and strokes, aligning with a preventive health strategy.

122. Psyllium Husk

Description:

Psyllium husk is a form of fiber made from the husks of the Plantago ovata plant's seeds. It is especially effective in lowering cholesterol levels and promoting heart health.

Usage:

Take psyllium husk as directed on the package, typically one to two teaspoons mixed with water, once daily. It's most effective when incorporated into a diet low in saturated fats.

Benefits:

Regular consumption of psyllium husk can help reduce LDL cholesterol levels and promote a healthy cardiovascular system. Its ability to absorb water in the digestive system also aids in digestion and regular bowel movements, contributing to overall health maintenance.

123. Hearty Barley Soup

Description:

Enjoy a nutritious and heart-healthy Hearty Barley Soup, rich in fiber and beta-glucan to help lower cholesterol levels and promote cardiovascular health.

Ingredients:

- 1 cup pearled barley
- 6 cups vegetable or chicken broth
- 1 onion, chopped
- 2 carrots, diced
- 2 stalks celery, diced
- 3 cloves garlic, minced
- 1 cup chopped tomatoes
- 2 cups spinach leaves
- Salt and pepper to taste
- Optional: herbs like thyme or parsley for added flavor

Preparation Steps:

1. Rinse barley under cold water until water is clear.
2. In a large pot, sauté onions, carrots, celery, and garlic until onions are translucent.
3. Add the rinsed barley and broth, bring to a boil.
4. Reduce heat and simmer for 30 minutes or until barley is tender.
5. Add chopped tomatoes and spinach, cook for an additional 5 minutes.
6. Season with salt, pepper, and optional herbs.

Usage:

Serve this wholesome soup as a main course or a hearty side dish to complement your meals.

Benefits:

This soup not only provides a comforting meal but also contributes to heart health by lowering cholesterol. The fiber in barley helps in digestive health, while the vegetables add essential nutrients and antioxidants, enhancing overall wellness.

124. Spirulina Smoothie

Description:

Boost your heart health with this nutrient-packed Spirulina Smoothie, rich in proteins, vitamins, and minerals that help lower blood pressure and cholesterol.

Ingredients:

- 1 teaspoon spirulina powder
- 1 banana
- 1 cup fresh spinach
- 1/2 cup unsweetened almond milk
- 1/2 apple, cored and sliced
- 1 tablespoon flaxseeds
- 1 teaspoon honey (optional)

Preparation Steps:

1. Place all ingredients in a blender.
2. Blend on high until smooth and creamy.
3. Taste and adjust sweetness with honey if desired.

Usage:

Enjoy this Spirulina Smoothie as a healthy breakfast or a refreshing snack to aid your cardiovascular health.

Benefits:

Spirulina is celebrated for its cardiovascular benefits, including lowering blood pressure and cholesterol. This smoothie combines spirulina with other heart-healthy ingredients like flaxseeds and spinach, enhancing overall wellness while providing a delicious way to support heart health.

Description:

Apple cider vinegar is praised for its heart-health

benefits, particularly in balancing cholesterol levels and enhancing cardiovascular health.

Ingredients:

- 2 tablespoons apple cider vinegar
- 1 tablespoon honey
- 1 cup warm water
- A squeeze of fresh lemon juice (optional)

Preparation Steps:

1. Combine apple cider vinegar and honey in warm water.
2. Add a squeeze of fresh lemon juice for extra flavor and antioxidants.
3. Stir well until the honey dissolves completely.

Usage:

Drink once daily, preferably in the morning on an empty stomach, to support heart health and maintain balanced cholesterol levels.

Benefits:

Regular consumption of this tonic can help improve lipid profiles and contribute to overall cardiovascular wellness, aligning with a heart-healthy diet.

PAIN RELIEF REMEDIES

125. Willow Bark Tea

Description:

Willow bark, known as "nature's aspirin," contains salicin which helps relieve pain and reduce inflammation effectively.

Ingredients:

- 1-2 teaspoons dried willow bark
- 1 cup boiling water

Preparation Steps:

1. Place dried willow bark in a tea infuser or directly in a cup.
2. Pour boiling water over the bark.
3. Steep for 10-15 minutes then strain if necessary.

Usage:

Drink this tea up to twice a day when experiencing pain such as headaches, back pain, or arthritis-related discomfort.

Benefits:

Willow bark tea offers a natural way to alleviate pain without the gastrointestinal side effects often associated with synthetic aspirin.

126. Turmeric Curcumin Tea

Description:

Turmeric, rich in curcumin, is highly effective in reducing joint pain and inflammation thanks to its potent anti-inflammatory properties.

Ingredients:

- 1 teaspoon turmeric powder
- 1/2 teaspoon black pepper (to enhance absorption)
- 1 teaspoon honey (optional, for taste)
- 1 cup water

Preparation Steps:

1. Boil water and add turmeric and black pepper.
2. Simmer for 10 minutes.
3. Strain into a cup and add honey if desired.

Usage:

Drink once or twice daily to manage symptoms of inflammation and pain.

Benefits:

Turmeric curcumin tea can help reduce symptoms of arthritis and other inflammatory conditions, supporting overall joint health and mobility.

127. Homemade Capsaicin Cream

Description:

Craft your own capsaicin cream using chili peppers to reduce pain by temporarily blocking pain signals.

Ingredients:

- 1/4 cup coconut oil
- 1 teaspoon cayenne pepper powder
- 1/2 cup shea butter

Preparation Steps:

1. Melt coconut oil and shea butter over low heat.
2. Stir in cayenne pepper powder evenly.
3. Allow the mixture to cool slightly before pouring into a jar.
4. Let it set in a cool place until solid.

Usage:

Apply a small amount to affected areas, avoiding open wounds or sensitive skin.

Benefits:

Capsaicin cream can effectively manage joint and nerve pain by reducing the intensity of pain signals sent through the body.

128. DIY Arnica Gel

Description:

Create your own arnica gel for topical application to soothe sore muscles, reduce inflammation, and expedite healing of bruises.

Ingredients:

- 1/4 cup arnica-infused oil
- 1/8 cup aloe vera gel
- 1 teaspoon beeswax

Preparation Steps:

1. Gently heat the arnica-infused oil and beeswax together until the beeswax melts completely.
2. Remove from heat and stir in the aloe vera gel until fully integrated.
3. Pour the mixture into a container and allow it to cool and set.

Usage:

Apply a thin layer of the gel to the affected area with gentle rubbing. Use two to three times daily.

Benefits:

Arnica gel provides natural pain relief and reduces swelling in the affected areas, promoting faster recovery from bruises and muscle soreness.

129. CBD Oil

Description:

CBD oil is derived from the cannabis plant and is known for its ability to alleviate chronic pain and reduce inflammation without psychoactive effects.

Usage:

Apply topically to affected areas for localized relief, or ingest a few drops under the tongue for systemic benefits. Always follow the dosage recommendations provided on the product label.

Benefits:

CBD oil interacts with the body's endocannabinoid system to help modulate pain and inflammation, offering a natural approach to pain management. This aligns with a holistic health approach, emphasizing natural, plant-based treatments for chronic conditions.

130. Ginger Supplements

Description:

Ginger supplements harness the powerful anti-inflammatory properties of ginger root, making them an effective natural alternative to NSAIDs for pain management.

Usage:

Take ginger supplements according to the manufacturer's instructions, typically with meals to minimize any potential stomach discomfort.

Benefits:

Regular intake of ginger supplements can help reduce inflammation, alleviate pain, particularly in conditions like arthritis, and support overall digestive health. This approach supports a natural, non-pharmacological pathway to managing pain and inflammation, reflecting the principles of using food as medicine.

131. Omega-3 Rich Smoothie

Description:

This smoothie is packed with omega-3 fatty acids, which are essential for reducing inflammation and alleviating joint pain, particularly in inflammatory conditions like rheumatoid arthritis.

Ingredients:

- 1 banana
- 1/2 cup blueberries
- 1 tablespoon flaxseeds or chia seeds
- 1 cup spinach
- 1/2 avocado
- 1 cup almond milk or any other plant-based milk

Preparation Steps:

1. Place all ingredients in a blender.
2. Blend until smooth.
3. Serve chilled for a refreshing and anti-inflammatory boost.

Usage:

Enjoy this smoothie daily, especially in the morning, to incorporate a healthy dose of omega-3s into your diet, which can help manage inflammation and pain.

Benefits:

The ingredients in this smoothie offer a synergistic blend of nutrients that promote joint health and overall well-being. Omega-3 fatty acids from flaxseeds, chia seeds, and avocado help reduce inflammation, while the antioxidants in blueberries and the vitamins in spinach support a healthy immune system.

132. Magnesium-Rich Banana and Spinach Smoothie

Description:

This smoothie combines banana and spinach, two magnesium-rich foods, to help relax tense muscles and alleviate symptoms like headaches and migraines.

Ingredients:

- 1 ripe banana
- 1 cup fresh spinach
- 1 tablespoon pumpkin seeds
- 1 cup unsweetened almond milk
- 1 tablespoon honey (optional)

Preparation Steps:

1. Place the banana, spinach, pumpkin seeds, and almond milk in a blender.
2. Blend until smooth.

3. Add honey if desired for sweetness and blend again to mix.

Usage:

Drink this smoothie in the morning or whenever you feel muscle tension or the onset of a headache.

Benefits:

Bananas and spinach provide a healthy dose of magnesium, which is essential for muscle relaxation and nerve function. Pumpkin seeds add additional magnesium and other minerals, enhancing the smoothie's ability to soothe muscle cramps and manage headache symptoms.

133. Lavender Essential Oil Massage Blend

Description:

Lavender essential oil is renowned for its ability to alleviate muscle tension and pain through its calming and relaxing properties.

Ingredients:

- 5 drops of lavender essential oil
- 1 tablespoon of sweet almond oil

Preparation Steps:

1. Mix the lavender essential oil with sweet almond oil in a small container.
2. Stir well to ensure the oils are thoroughly blended.

Usage:

Apply the oil blend to areas of muscle tension or pain and massage gently. Use before bedtime to enhance relaxation and improve sleep quality.

Benefits:

Lavender oil's soothing scent helps to calm the mind and reduce stress, while its anti-inflammatory properties help relieve pain and muscle tension.

Sweet almond oil serves as a carrier, facilitating the absorption of lavender oil and nourishing the skin with vitamins.

134. Peppermint Essential Oil Remedy

Description:

Peppermint oil, known for its cooling and soothing effects, is effective in relieving headache symptoms.

Ingredients:

- Peppermint essential oil
- Carrier oil (such as coconut or jojoba oil)

Preparation Steps:

Mix a few drops of peppermint essential oil with a teaspoon of carrier oil.

Usage:

Massage the mixture gently onto the temples and neck area when experiencing a headache.

Benefits:

The menthol in peppermint oil helps to relax muscles and ease pain, providing quick relief from headaches.

135. Boswellia Serrata Remedy

Description:

Boswellia serrata, often used in traditional medicine, is recognized for its anti-inflammatory properties, especially beneficial for those suffering from osteoarthritis.

Ingredients:

- Boswellia serrata extract

Usage:

Take Boswellia serrata supplements as directed, typically in capsule form.

Benefits:

Regular use of Boswellia can significantly reduce joint pain and inflammation, aiding mobility and enhancing quality of life for individuals with osteoarthritis.

136. Valerian Root Remedy

Description:

Valerian root is valued for its calming effects and ability to ease muscle and menstrual pain due to its sedative and antispasmodic properties.

Ingredients:

▫ Dried valerian root

Preparation Steps:

1. Boil water
2. Add about 1 teaspoon of dried valerian root per cup of hot water
3. Steep for 10 to 15 minutes
4. Strain the mixture

Usage:

Drink valerian root tea an hour before bedtime or during menstrual periods to relieve pain and improve sleep.

Benefits:

Regular consumption can help manage pain and promote relaxation, reducing the need for conventional pain relievers.

137. White Willow Tea Remedy

Description:

White willow bark is known as a natural analgesic, effective for easing lower back pain and symptoms of osteoarthritis.

Ingredients:

▫ Dried white willow bark

Preparation Steps:

1. Boil water
2. Add 1 to 2 teaspoons of dried white willow bark per cup of hot water
3. Simmer for 10 to 15 minutes
4. Strain the tea

Usage:

Consume a cup of white willow bark tea when experiencing pain to utilize its salicin content, which the body converts into pain-relieving salicylic acid.

Benefits:

White willow tea offers a gentle approach to pain management, reducing dependence on synthetic pain medication while providing effective relief from chronic pain and inflammation.

138. Devil's Claw Remedy

Description:

Devil's Claw is a herb recognized for its ability to reduce inflammation and alleviate pain, particularly in the back and joints.

Ingredients:

▫ Dried Devil's Claw root

Preparation Steps:

1. Boil water
2. Add 1 teaspoon of dried Devil's Claw root per cup of water
3. Simmer for about 20 minutes
4. Strain the liquid

Usage:

Drink a cup of Devil's Claw tea up to two times a day

to manage symptoms of pain and inflammation, especially in conditions like osteoarthritis and back pain.

Benefits:

Devil's Claw tea can serve as a natural alternative to conventional anti-inflammatories, offering relief from pain without the common side effects of over-the-counter medications.

139. MSM Supplement Remedy

Description:

MSM, or Methylsulfonylmethane, is a sulfur-containing compound known for its ability to decrease joint pain and inflammation, as well as enhance skin health.

Ingredients:

- MSM powder or capsules

Preparation Steps:

Purchase pure MSM powder or capsules from a reputable health store.

If using powder, mix the recommended amount (usually around 1-2 grams) with water or juice.

Usage:

Consume MSM according to the package instructions, typically once or twice daily, to support joint and skin health.

Benefits:

Regular intake of MSM supplements can help reduce chronic pain and stiffness associated with joint disorders such as arthritis, promote skin healing and elasticity, and improve overall inflammatory responses in the body.

140. Eucalyptus Essential Oil Remedy

Description:

Eucalyptus essential oil is celebrated for its analgesic properties that aid in alleviating pain and soothing tension headaches.

Ingredients:

- Eucalyptus essential oil
- Diffuser or a bowl of hot water

Preparation Steps:

1. For diffusion: Add a few drops of eucalyptus oil to your diffuser and turn it on according to the machine's instructions.

2. For steam inhalation: Add 3-4 drops of eucalyptus oil to a bowl of boiling water.

Usage:

Inhale the vapor deeply to help clear the head and relieve tension. Use as needed when experiencing headaches or when you need relief from nasal congestion.

Benefits:

Eucalyptus oil not only helps to clear sinuses and relieve headache pain but also promotes relaxation of tense facial muscles often associated with headaches and stress.

141. Kratom Remedy

Description:

Kratom is recognized for its significant pain-relief capabilities, particularly effective for individuals dealing with chronic pain. It should be used responsibly, considering legal restrictions in some regions.

Ingredients:

- Kratom leaves (dried or fresh)
- Hot water

Preparation Steps:

1. Boil water and add kratom leaves.

2. Allow to steep for 5-10 minutes, depending on desired strength.

3. Strain the mixture to remove the leaves.

Usage:

Consume the tea once it's cool enough to drink. It's important to start with a small amount to assess tolerance and effect.

Benefits:

Kratom can offer profound relief from chronic pain, potentially enhancing quality of life. However, it's important to use this herb under the guidance of a healthcare provider due to its potent effects and legal considerations.

142. Bromelain Pineapple Smoothie

Description:

Bromelain, extracted from pineapple, is renowned for its effectiveness in alleviating inflammation and pain, especially useful after surgeries or physical injuries.

Ingredients:

- 1 cup fresh pineapple, chopped
- 1/2 banana
- 1/2 cup Greek yogurt
- 1 teaspoon honey
- Ice cubes

Preparation Steps:

1. Combine pineapple, banana, Greek yogurt, and honey in a blender.

2. Add ice cubes to preference.

3. Blend until smooth.

Usage:

Enjoy this smoothie once a day, particularly after physical activities or post-surgery, to aid in recovery and reduce inflammation.

Benefits:

Bromelain's anti-inflammatory properties help speed up recovery by reducing swelling and pain. This smoothie not only delivers these benefits but also provides a delicious, refreshing way to support your health.

143. Hot Chili Pepper Liniment

Description:

Capsaicin, derived from hot chili peppers, is utilized topically to diminish pain signals by desensitizing nerve endings, offering relief from various types of pain.

Ingredients:

- 2 tablespoons of chili powder
- 1/2 cup olive oil
- 1/4 cup grated beeswax

Preparation Steps:

1. Gently heat the olive oil in a saucepan.

2. Stir in the chili powder and allow to infuse on low heat for about 10 minutes.

3. Add grated beeswax and stir until fully melted.

4. Strain the mixture through a fine sieve or cheesecloth into a container.

5. Let the liniment cool until it solidifies.

Usage:

Apply a small amount to the affected area, avoiding open wounds or sensitive skin. Use gloves to prevent irritation to your hands.

Benefits:

This liniment provides localized pain relief by interfering with pain signals to the brain, making it beneficial for conditions like arthritis, muscle strains, and back pain.

144. Comfrey Cream

Description:

Comfrey cream is utilized topically to accelerate healing in muscle sprains, joint pain, and bruises due to its high allantoin content, which stimulates cell growth and repair.

Ingredients:

- 1/4 cup dried comfrey leaves
- 1/2 cup coconut oil
- 1/4 cup shea butter
- 2 tablespoons beeswax

Preparation Steps:

1. Infuse the comfrey leaves in coconut oil over low heat for 30 minutes.
2. Strain the leaves and return the oil to the heat.
3. Add shea butter and beeswax to the infused oil, stirring until fully melted.
4. Pour the mixture into jars and allow to cool and set.

Usage:

Apply the cream to the affected area 2-3 times a day, massaging gently.

Benefits:

Comfrey cream supports the healing process of soft tissue injuries and reduces inflammation and pain, making it a valuable remedy for natural pain relief.

145. Acupuncture and Acupressure

Description:

Acupuncture and acupressure are traditional Chinese medicinal practices that involve stimulating specific points on the body to enhance health and alleviate pain.

Usage:

These techniques are commonly used for pain relief, stress reduction, and overall wellness improvement. Acupuncture involves the insertion of fine needles at key points, while acupressure uses gentle to firm finger pressure.

Benefits:

Both methods are effective for managing various types of pain, including chronic pain and headaches. They can also help reduce stress and anxiety, improve sleep patterns, and enhance circulation, contributing to better overall health and well-being.

146. Rosemary Essential Oil

Description:

Rosemary essential oil is renowned for its pain-relieving properties and its ability to stimulate blood circulation, aligning with the Outlive philosophy of using natural remedies for health enhancement.

Usage:

Apply the oil topically after diluting it with a carrier oil, or use it in aromatherapy diffusers. It can be massaged into affected areas to alleviate muscle pain or inhaled to reduce headaches.

Benefits:

Rosemary oil is beneficial for reducing muscle tension and pain, promoting better circulation—a key aspect of maintaining vitality as emphasized in the Outlive approach. Its invigorating scent also helps to enhance mental clarity and reduce fatigue, supporting overall cognitive health.

147. Akuamma Seed Pain Relief Tincture

Description:

Akuamma seeds, traditionally used in African medicine, contain the alkaloid akuammine, known for its potent analgesic properties.

Ingredients:

- Akuamma seeds
- High-proof alcohol (such as vodka or everclear)
- Dark glass bottle with dropper

Preparation Steps:

1. Crush the akuamma seeds into a fine powder.
2. Fill one-third of the dark glass bottle with the powdered akuamma seeds.
3. Pour high-proof alcohol into the bottle until the seeds are completely submerged.
4. Seal the bottle tightly and store in a cool, dark place for 4 to 6 weeks, shaking the bottle every few days.
5. After the infusion period, strain the tincture through a fine mesh sieve or cheesecloth into another dark glass bottle. Press or squeeze to extract as much liquid as possible.

Usage:

Administer 1-2 droppers of the tincture under the tongue, up to three times a day for pain relief. Hold under the tongue for 30 seconds before swallowing for best absorption.

Benefits:

This tincture harnesses the analgesic effects of akuamma seeds to help reduce pain. It can be particularly effective for managing chronic pain conditions, aligning with the Outlive philosophy of utilizing traditional remedies alongside modern practices for optimal health and longevity.

148. Clove Oil Dental Pain Reliever

Description:

Clove oil is renowned for its powerful analgesic and anti-inflammatory properties, making it highly effective for dental pain relief when applied topically.

Ingredients:

- Clove essential oil
- Carrier oil (such as coconut oil or olive oil)

Preparation Steps:

1. Mix 1 part clove essential oil with 10 parts carrier oil to dilute the essential oil and prevent irritation.
2. Store the mixture in a small, dark glass bottle to maintain its potency.

Usage:

Apply a small amount of the diluted clove oil mixture directly onto the gums around the painful area using a cotton swab or your fingertip. Use up to three times a day as needed for pain relief.

Benefits:

Clove oil contains eugenol, a natural anesthetic, which provides rapid relief from dental pain and reduces inflammation. Its antiseptic properties also help prevent infection, aligning with holistic approaches to health maintenance by using natural, minimally processed remedies.

149. Kava Kava Muscle Relaxant

Description:

Kava kava is widely used for its calming effects that help relieve muscle pain and promote overall relaxation.

Ingredients:

- Dried kava kava root

Preparation Steps:

1. Purchase high-quality dried kava kava root.
2. Grind the root into a fine powder using a coffee

grinder or mortar and pestle.

3. For a traditional preparation, mix the ground kava with cold water in a bowl. Use about one tablespoon of powder per cup of water.

4. Knead and squeeze the mixture in a cloth bag or strainer for several minutes to extract the kavalactones into the water.

5. Strain the liquid to remove any remaining solids.

Usage:

Drink a small cup of the prepared kava kava beverage to experience muscle relaxation and mental calming. Do not exceed two cups per day to avoid potential side effects.

Benefits:

Kava kava acts on the nervous system to induce relaxation without impairing cognitive function, making it an excellent remedy for stress-related muscle tension. It's particularly useful in promoting better sleep, which is essential for muscle recovery and stress relief, echoing the holistic approach of enhancing body wellness through natural means.

SKIN AND HAIR CARE REMEDIES

150. Aloe Vera Gel Recipe

Description:

Aloe vera gel is celebrated for its exceptional soothing and healing properties, making it ideal for treating skin irritations like sunburns, hydrating the skin, and aiding in the repair of minor cuts and scrapes.

Ingredients:

▫ Fresh aloe vera leaf

Preparation Steps:

1. Select a thick aloe vera leaf from an aloe plant.

2. Cut the leaf from the base using a sharp knife.

3. Stand the leaf upright in a cup for a few minutes to allow the yellow sap (aloe latex) to drain out. This sap can be irritating to the skin.

4. Wash the leaf thoroughly.

5. Carefully peel off the skin from one side of the leaf to expose the clear gel.

6. Scoop out the gel using a spoon or knife and place it in a clean bowl.

7. For a smoother gel, blend the scooped gel for a few seconds until it is frothy and even.

Usage:

Apply the gel directly to the affected area of the skin. You can store the remainder in a sealed container in the refrigerator for up to one week.

Benefits:

Aloe vera gel contains compounds that are anti-inflammatory, which can reduce skin inflammation and speed healing. Its hydrating properties also help to retain moisture in the skin, promoting a healthier, more vibrant complexion. This aligns well with the holistic approaches to skin care, emphasizing natural, toxin-free ingredients for long-term health benefits.

151. Coconut Oil Hair Treatment

Description:

Coconut oil is a natural emollient, perfect for moisturizing hair and reducing protein loss in damaged strands, making it a staple in natural hair care routines.

Ingredients:

▫ Virgin coconut oil

Preparation Steps:

1. Measure out a small amount of virgin coconut oil, depending on hair length and thickness.

2. If solid, gently warm the coconut oil in a microwave-safe container or in a double boiler until it melts. Ensure it is warm but not hot.

Usage:

1. Apply the melted coconut oil to dry or damp hair, starting from the midsection and working towards the ends. For deeper conditioning, massage the oil into the scalp.

2. Cover hair with a shower cap and let the oil sit for at least 30 minutes or overnight for intensive moisturization.

3. Wash hair with shampoo and optionally condition after to remove excess oil.

Benefits:

Coconut oil not only moisturizes and strengthens hair but also provides essential proteins required for nourishing damaged hair. Its ability to penetrate the hair shaft makes it ideal for reducing protein loss in hair — a common issue for those with chemically treated or frequently styled hair. This aligns with the holistic approach of nurturing body and beauty with natural, minimally processed substances.

152. Tea Tree Oil Scalp and Skin Treatment

Description:

Tea tree oil is renowned for its potent antibacterial and antifungal properties, effectively treating acne, dandruff, and scalp irritations.

Ingredients:

- Tea tree essential oil

- Carrier oil (such as coconut oil or jojoba oil)

Preparation Steps:

1. Mix a few drops of tea tree essential oil with a tablespoon of carrier oil to dilute it, ensuring it is safe for direct skin application.

2. Stir well to ensure the oils are thoroughly combined.

Usage:

For acne: Apply the oil mixture directly to clean skin with a cotton swab, targeting affected areas. Use sparingly — tea tree oil is potent.

For scalp treatment: Massage the oil mixture into the scalp before bedtime. Leave it overnight for maximum effect and wash out with shampoo in the morning.

For dandruff: Apply the oil mixture to the scalp and let sit for about 30 minutes before washing your hair as usual.

Benefits:

Using tea tree oil can significantly reduce skin and scalp infections due to its natural antimicrobial properties. It helps clear up acne, soothes itchy scalps, reduces dandruff, and can prevent fungal infections. Incorporating this natural remedy supports a healthier, more balanced approach to personal care, reflecting the principles of maintaining cleanliness and health through natural, effective solutions.

153. Argan Oil Hair and Skin Nourisher

Description:

Argan oil, known as 'liquid gold,' is packed with vitamin E and essential fatty acids, making it excellent for hair and skin care.

Usage:

For hair: Work a few drops into damp or dry hair to smooth frizz and add shine.

For skin: Apply directly to the skin or mix with your daily moisturizer for extra hydration.

Benefits:

Argan oil deeply hydrates and nourishes the skin and hair, restores elasticity, and gives a natural boost of moisture and shine, promoting a healthier appearance.

154. Jojoba Oil Hydration Solution

Description:

Jojoba oil closely mimics the skin's natural sebum, making it an excellent moisturizer for both skin and hair without clogging pores.

Usage:

For skin: Apply a few drops to clean, damp skin as a moisturizer.

For hair: Use as a pre-shampoo scalp treatment or apply to damp hair to seal moisture and enhance shine.

Benefits:

Jojoba oil provides deep hydration, regulating skin's oil production and improving hair softness and shine, making it ideal for daily use.

155. Shea Butter

Description:

Shea butter is celebrated for its rich conditioning qualities, ideal for deeply softening the skin and rejuvenating damaged hair.

Usage:

Use it as a body moisturizer after bathing or apply it to hair as a leave-in conditioner to heal dry and brittle strands.

Benefits:

Shea butter infuses the skin and hair with moisture, helps repair damage, and provides a protective barrier to lock in hydration, enhancing both skin and hair health.

156. Apple Cider Vinegar

Description:

Apple cider vinegar is renowned for its ability to balance the skin and hair's pH, enhancing their texture and shine.

Ingredients:

- Apple cider vinegar
- Water

Preparation Steps:

1. Mix one part apple cider vinegar with three parts water in a clean bottle.

2. Shake well to ensure it is thoroughly mixed.

Usage:

Use as a facial toner by applying with a cotton pad, or as a hair rinse after shampooing. Apply to the scalp and hair, leave for a few minutes, then rinse out.

Benefits:

This diluted apple cider vinegar solution helps to reduce dandruff, promote shiny hair, and restore natural pH levels of the skin, preventing excessive oiliness and improving overall skin health.

157. Baking Soda

Description:

Baking soda serves as a versatile ingredient for skin and hair care, acting as a gentle exfoliant and effective scalp cleanser.

Ingredients:

- Baking soda
- Water

Preparation Steps:

1. Mix baking soda with a small amount of water to create a paste.

2. Stir until the mixture reaches a spreadable consistency.

Usage:

For skin, apply the paste to your face with gentle circular motions, then rinse with warm water. For hair, massage the paste into your scalp before rinsing thoroughly during your shower.

Benefits:

Using baking soda as a scrub can help remove dead skin cells and cleanse pores, leading to clearer and smoother skin. As a scalp cleanser, it removes product buildup, leaving your hair clean and refreshed.

158. Castor Oil

Description:

Castor oil is a natural oil that promotes hair growth and is used to thicken hair, eyelashes, and eyebrows effectively.

Usage:

Apply a small amount of castor oil to the scalp, hair, or eyebrows using a clean brush or fingertips. For eyelashes, use a clean mascara wand or a cotton swab. Apply preferably before bedtime.

Benefits:

Regular application of castor oil can enhance hair thickness and accelerate growth due to its rich content of ricinoleic acid and omega-6 essential fatty acids. It also moisturizes and can help prevent hair breakage and loss.

159. Lavender Essential Oil Scalp Treatment

Description:

Lavender essential oil is celebrated for its calming effects on the skin and its ability to soothe scalp irritations and promote healthy hair growth.

Ingredients:

- 5 drops of lavender essential oil
- 2 tablespoons of coconut oil

Preparation Steps:

1. Warm the coconut oil slightly until it is liquid.
2. Add the lavender essential oil to the warmed coconut oil and mix well.

Usage:

Massage the oil mixture into your scalp and leave it on for at least 30 minutes or overnight for deeper conditioning. Wash out using your regular shampoo routine.

Benefits:

This scalp treatment helps to reduce inflammation and irritation, soothes dry and itchy scalp, and enhances blood circulation to the scalp which can promote healthier hair growth. Lavender's natural antiseptic and antifungal properties also help to keep the scalp healthy.

160. Rosehip Oil Remedy

Description:

Rosehip oil is rich in vitamins A and C, making it excellent for skin regeneration and improving skin elasticity. It is also known for its ability to reduce scars and fine lines.

Usage:

Apply 2-3 drops of rosehip oil directly to the face or affected area twice daily, morning and night.

Benefits:

Regular application of rosehip oil can enhance skin rejuvenation, help fade age spots, and improve firmness by promoting collagen production. It's particularly effective for reducing the appearance of scars and fine lines, making it a valuable addition to a skincare routine.

161. Peppermint Oil Remedy

Description:

Peppermint oil invigorates the scalp, promotes hair growth, and provides relief from skin irritation, making it a versatile addition to beauty and health routines.

Ingredients:

- Peppermint essential oil
- Carrier oil (such as jojoba or coconut oil)

Preparation Steps:

1. Mix 2-3 drops of peppermint essential oil with a tablespoon of carrier oil to dilute.
2. Store the mixture in a dark glass bottle to preserve its potency.

Usage:

1. Massage the oil blend into the scalp for a few minutes to stimulate circulation.
2. Apply to irritated skin areas for soothing effects.

Benefits:

Peppermint oil's cooling sensation helps calm irritation, reduce redness, and alleviate itchiness on the skin. When used on the scalp, it stimulates blood flow, which can promote healthier, faster hair growth.

162. Honey & Cinnamon Acne Treatment

Description:

Combining honey's natural antibacterial properties with the anti-inflammatory benefits of cinnamon creates a potent remedy for acne.

Ingredients:

- 2 tablespoons raw, organic honey
- 1 teaspoon ground cinnamon

Preparation Steps:

1. Mix the honey and cinnamon together until you achieve a consistent paste.
2. Ensure the mixture is thoroughly combined for maximum effectiveness.

Usage:

Apply the mixture directly to clean, dry skin, focusing on areas with acne. Leave the mask on for 10-15 minutes before rinsing off with warm water. Use up to twice a week for best results.

Benefits:

This remedy helps fight bacterial infections in the skin and reduces inflammation. Honey moisturizes without clogging pores, while cinnamon enhances circulation and exfoliates, promoting a healthier skin surface and reducing pimples.

163. Green Tea Skin Revitalizer

Description:

Green tea is renowned for its antioxidant-rich composition, making it an excellent choice for a skin revitalizer to combat signs of aging and environmental damage.

Ingredients:

- 2 tablespoons of loose organic green tea leaves
- 1 cup of boiling water

Preparation Steps:

1. Steep the green tea leaves in boiling water for 10 minutes to fully extract the antioxidants.
2. Strain the leaves and let the tea cool to room temperature.
3. Pour the tea into a clean spray bottle for easy application.

Usage:

Spray the cooled green tea onto clean, dry skin. Use daily in the morning or evening, and under sunscreen for added daytime protection.

Benefits:

Green tea's antioxidants neutralize skin-damaging free radicals, improving skin elasticity and reducing signs of aging. Its anti-inflammatory properties soothe redness and irritation, enhancing skin clarity.

164. Avocado Skin and Hair Nourisher

Description:

Avocado is packed with essential fatty acids and vitamins, making it an ideal natural enhancer for both skin and hair, providing deep moisturization and conditioning.

Ingredients:

1. 1 ripe avocado
2. 1 tablespoon of honey (for skin application)
3. 2 tablespoons of olive oil (for hair application)

Preparation Steps:

1. Mash the ripe avocado into a smooth paste.
2. Mix in honey for a skin mask or olive oil for a hair conditioner.

Usage:

For skin: Apply the avocado and honey mixture to your face, leave on for 15 minutes, then rinse with warm water.

For hair: Work the avocado and olive oil mixture into damp hair, leave for 20 minutes, then wash out with shampoo.

Benefits:

Avocado deeply moisturizes the skin, leaving it soft and supple, while the hair treatment reduces dryness and adds shine. Its vitamins and fatty acids help rejuvenate and protect, maintaining healthy skin and hair as part of a longevity-focused regimen.

165. Cucumber Soothing Eye Treatment

Description:

Cucumber is celebrated for its hydrating and anti-inflammatory properties, making it perfect for soothing puffy eyes and refreshing the skin.

Ingredients:

- 1 fresh cucumber

Preparation Steps:

1. Slice the cucumber into thin rounds.
2. Chill the slices in the refrigerator for enhanced soothing effects.

Usage:

Place the chilled cucumber slices over your eyes and relax for 10-15 minutes. Use daily or whenever the eyes feel particularly tired or puffy.

Benefits:

Cucumber slices help reduce eye puffiness and soothe tired eyes due to their high water content and anti-inflammatory properties. Regular use can help maintain a refreshed and youthful appearance around the eyes, aligning with longevity practices that emphasize natural, preventive skin care.

166. Zinc Oxide Natural Sunscreen

Description:

Zinc oxide is a key ingredient in natural sunscreen products, providing broad-spectrum protection against UVA and UVB rays without the use of harmful chemicals.

Ingredients:

- 1/4 cup zinc oxide powder
- 1/4 cup shea butter

- 1/4 cup coconut oil
- 1 tablespoon beeswax

Preparation Steps:

1. Melt the shea butter, coconut oil, and beeswax together in a double boiler.

2. Remove from heat and let the mixture cool slightly before stirring in the zinc oxide powder until well combined.

Usage:

Apply liberally to exposed skin before going outdoors, reapplying every two hours, or after swimming or sweating.

Benefits:

This natural sunscreen provides a physical barrier against harmful UV rays, reducing sun damage and premature aging. Zinc oxide's gentle nature makes it suitable for all skin types, supporting skin health and longevity without chemical exposure.

167. Almond Oil Skin and Hair Enhancer

Description:

Almond oil is highly beneficial for both skin and hair, known for its ability to soften skin, clear complexion, impart a glow, condition hair, and improve scalp health.

Usage:

For skin: Massage a few drops of almond oil into the face and body as needed.

For hair: Apply almond oil to the scalp and hair, leaving it on for at least 30 minutes before shampooing.

Benefits:

Almond oil nourishes the skin, enhancing elasticity and giving it a healthy glow while clearing the complexion. It hydrates the hair, reduces scalp

irritation, and promotes stronger, shinier hair. Regular use supports overall dermatological health and aligns with longevity practices by nourishing the body naturally.

168. Sulfur Acne Treatment

Description:

Sulfur is an effective ingredient in natural acne treatments, known for its ability to dry out the skin's surface and absorb excess oils that contribute to acne formation.

Ingredients:

- Pure micronized sulfur
- Distilled water

Preparation Steps:

Mix 1 tablespoon of micronized sulfur with 2 tablespoons of distilled water to form a paste.

Usage:

Apply the sulfur paste directly to the affected areas of the skin. Let it sit for 10-15 minutes before rinsing off with lukewarm water.

Benefits:

Sulfur's drying effect reduces skin oiliness and helps clear up acne blemishes. Its antibacterial properties also prevent future breakouts, making it a valuable treatment for maintaining clear skin and supporting a healthy complexion.

169. Clay Detoxifying Mask

Description:

Clay, particularly Bentonite or Kaolin, is highly effective for drawing out impurities and absorbing excess oil from the skin, making it ideal for detoxifying facial masks.

Ingredients:

- 2 tablespoons of Bentonite or Kaolin clay

□ Water or rose water

Preparation Steps:

1. Mix the clay with enough water or rose water to form a smooth paste.

Usage:

Apply the clay mask evenly over the face, avoiding the eye area. Allow it to dry for about 10-15 minutes before rinsing off with warm water.

Benefits:

This clay mask purifies the skin by removing impurities and absorbing oil, which helps prevent acne and promotes a clearer complexion. Regular use can refine pores and enhance skin texture, contributing to a healthier and more radiant appearance.

170. Oatmeal Soothing Skin Treatment

Description:

Oatmeal is celebrated for its soothing properties, making it an excellent choice for natural remedies targeting irritated skin or eczema.

Ingredients:

□ 1/2 cup of colloidal oatmeal (finely ground oats)

□ Warm water

Preparation Steps:

Mix colloidal oatmeal with warm water to create a thick, spreadable paste.

Usage:

Apply the oatmeal paste directly to the affected areas. Leave it on the skin for about 15-20 minutes before rinsing off gently with lukewarm water.

Benefits:

Oatmeal calms skin irritation and reduces inflammation, making it ideal for soothing eczema and other skin irritations. Its moisturizing

properties also help to restore the skin's natural barrier.

171. Avocado & Almond Vitamin E Rich Facial Mask

Description:

Leveraging the natural Vitamin E content in avocado and almond oil, this facial mask nourishes and protects the skin, enhancing its ability to repair and resist damage from free radicals.

Ingredients:

□ 1 ripe avocado

□ 1 tablespoon almond oil

□ 1 teaspoon honey (optional for additional moisturizing)

Preparation Steps:

1. Mash the ripe avocado into a smooth paste.

2. Mix in almond oil and honey until the mixture is well combined.

Usage:

Apply the mask evenly over the face, leaving it on for about 20 minutes. Wash off with warm water and pat dry. Use once a week for best results.

Benefits:

This mask combines the antioxidant power of Vitamin E with the hydrating properties of avocado and almond oil, providing deep nourishment and protection against environmental damage. Regular use can improve skin elasticity, moisture retention, and overall skin health, contributing to a rejuvenated complexion.

172. Sea Salt Exfoliating Scrub

Description:

Sea salt is an excellent exfoliant for removing dead skin cells and improving circulation, making it a vital component in natural skincare routines for rejuvenated, smooth skin.

Ingredients:

- 1/4 cup fine sea salt
- 1/4 cup olive oil or coconut oil
- Optional: 5-10 drops of essential oil (like lavender or peppermint for additional benefits and fragrance)

Preparation Steps:

1. Mix the sea salt with your choice of oil until fully integrated.
2. Add essential oil if desired and stir to combine.

Usage:

Gently massage the scrub into damp skin in a circular motion, focusing on rough areas like elbows and knees. Rinse off with warm water. Use once or twice a week to avoid over-exfoliation.

Benefits:

This scrub sloughs off dead skin cells and improves circulation, promoting healthier skin regeneration. The oils moisturize and soothe the skin, leaving it soft and radiant with each use.

173. Neem Oil Therapeutic Treatment

Description:

Neem oil is renowned for its antiseptic, antifungal, and anti-inflammatory properties, making it a powerful treatment for various skin conditions and an effective solution for maintaining scalp health.

Ingredients:

- Pure neem oil
- Carrier oil (like coconut or jojoba oil) for dilution

Preparation Steps:

1. Dilute neem oil with the carrier oil in a 1:10 ratio to ensure it is gentle on the skin and scalp.

Usage:

For skin: Apply the diluted neem oil to affected areas using a cotton ball, leaving it on for up to 20 minutes before rinsing.

For scalp: Massage the diluted oil into the scalp, leave for 30 minutes, then shampoo thoroughly.

ENERGY BOOSTERS

174. Matcha Green Tea Energy Elixir

Description:

Matcha green tea is loaded with antioxidants and offers a unique blend of L-theanine and caffeine, providing a smooth, sustained energy boost and improved focus without the common jitteriness associated with coffee.

Ingredients:

- 1-2 teaspoons of high-quality matcha green tea powder
- Hot water (not boiling, to preserve nutrients)

Preparation Steps:

1. Sift the matcha powder into a cup to avoid clumps.
2. Add hot water and whisk vigorously in a zigzag motion until the tea is frothy.

Usage:

Drink a cup of matcha green tea in the morning or early afternoon for a natural energy boost and enhanced mental clarity throughout the day.

Benefits:

Matcha increases energy levels and concentration over several hours, unlike the short spikes provided by traditional coffee. Its high antioxidant content also supports overall health, making it a valuable addition to a longevity-focused lifestyle.

175. Maca Root Energy Booster

Description:

Maca root powder is recognized as a natural energizer, known for enhancing stamina and endurance when added to daily meals like smoothies or breakfast bowls.

Ingredients:

1. 1 tablespoon maca root powder
2. Your choice of smoothie or breakfast bowl ingredients

Preparation Steps:

Incorporate maca root powder into your favorite smoothie recipe or sprinkle it over your breakfast bowl.

Usage:

Enjoy a maca-infused smoothie or breakfast bowl in the morning to kickstart your day with increased energy and improved endurance.

Benefits:

Maca root not only boosts energy levels but also helps balance hormones and improves overall vitality. Regular consumption can enhance physical and mental performance, supporting an active and energized lifestyle.

176. Coconut Water Hydration Boost

Description:

Coconut water is rich in essential electrolytes such as potassium and magnesium, making it an excellent choice for natural hydration and energy enhancement.

Ingredients:

▫ Pure coconut water

Preparation Steps:

Choose fresh, pure coconut water without added sugars or flavors for maximum benefits.

Usage:

Drink coconut water throughout the day or specifically after workouts to replenish hydration and electrolytes efficiently.

Benefits:

Coconut water naturally boosts energy levels and aids in hydration, thanks to its high electrolyte content. It is particularly beneficial for maintaining energy during physical activities and recovery, promoting overall health and vitality.

177. Spirulina Vitality Enhancer

Description:

Spirulina, a blue-green algae, is a nutrient powerhouse packed with protein, vitamins, and minerals, making it an excellent supplement for boosting energy levels and enhancing overall vitality.

Usage:

Incorporate spirulina powder into smoothies, juices, or water. Consume daily, preferably in the morning, to optimize energy levels throughout the day.

Benefits:

Spirulina supports sustained energy production due to its high concentrations of protein and essential nutrients. It also aids in immune function and can improve endurance and reduce fatigue, making it a valuable addition to a health-focused diet.

178. Rhodiola Rosea Stress Adaptation Tonic

Description:

Rhodiola Rosea, an adaptogen, aids the body in adapting to stress, enhancing energy, stamina, and mental capacity without the side effects commonly associated with stimulants.

Ingredients:

- Rhodiola Rosea extract (available in liquid, powder, or capsule form)

Preparation Steps:

1. Choose a high-quality Rhodiola Rosea supplement from a reputable source to ensure effectiveness and safety.

Usage:

Take Rhodiola Rosea according to package directions, typically once or twice daily, preferably in the morning and at midday to support energy and mental alertness throughout the day.

Benefits:

Rhodiola Rosea helps the body manage stress more effectively, boosting energy levels and mental performance. Its adaptogenic properties also support overall well-being and resilience, making it ideal for those with high-stress lifestyles.

179. Ginseng Energy Elixir

Description:

Ginseng is renowned for its ability to enhance overall energy and assist the body in coping with stress, making it a staple in herbal remedies for boosting vitality.

Ingredients:

- Ginseng root (available as fresh root, powder, or extract)

Preparation Steps:

1. If using fresh ginseng root, slice it thinly. For powder or extract, measure the recommended dosage.

Usage:

Incorporate ginseng into teas, smoothies, or consume directly if using extract. It's best taken in the morning or early afternoon to maximize its energizing effects without disturbing sleep.

Benefits:

Ginseng increases energy and improves stress resilience, enhancing both physical and mental performance. Regular use can help maintain high energy levels and support overall health, making it beneficial for those with demanding lifestyles.

180. Beetroot Juice Performance Enhancer

Description:

Beetroot juice is rich in nitrates, which improve blood flow and oxygenate the muscles, enhancing physical performance and boosting energy levels.

Ingredients:

- Fresh beetroots
- Water (optional for dilution)

Preparation Steps:

Juice fresh beetroots to extract the liquid. Dilute with water if the flavor is too strong.

Usage:

Drink a glass of beetroot juice about one to two hours before engaging in physical activity to benefit from increased stamina and energy.

Benefits:

The nitrates in beetroot juice enhance cardiovascular efficiency and muscle oxygenation, significantly improving endurance and energy during physical activities. This makes it an ideal natural supplement for athletes and those looking to boost their physical performance.

181. Chia Seed & Berry Energy Smoothie

Description:

This smoothie combines chia seeds with antioxidant-rich berries to create a nutritious, energizing drink. The fiber, protein, and omega-3 fatty acids in chia seeds work with the vitamins and minerals in berries to boost energy and overall health.

Ingredients:

- 2 tablespoons chia seeds
- 1 cup mixed berries (blueberries, strawberries, raspberries)
- 1 banana for sweetness
- 1 cup almond milk or any other plant-based milk
- 1 tablespoon honey (optional)

Preparation Steps:

1. Soak the chia seeds in a half cup of water for 20 minutes until they become gel-like.
2. Blend the soaked chia seeds with berries, banana, almond milk, and honey until smooth.

Usage:

Enjoy this smoothie in the morning or before a workout to fuel your body with sustained energy, thanks to the slow-release carbohydrates in the fruits and the high fiber content in chia seeds.

Benefits:

This smoothie enhances physical stamina and mental clarity throughout the day. Chia seeds provide a stable energy supply, while berries add essential nutrients and antioxidants that support immune function and reduce inflammation.

182. B Vitamin Complex Energy Boost Drink

Description:

B vitamins are crucial for energy production at the cellular level, helping convert dietary energy into ATP, the form of energy used by the body. This drink ensures you get a complete spectrum of B vitamins to support sustained energy throughout the day.

Ingredients:

- B vitamin complex supplement (in capsule or liquid form)
- 1 cup of orange juice (natural source of Vitamin C and folate)
- 1/2 cup of spinach (natural source of B vitamins and iron)

Preparation Steps:

1. Blend the orange juice and spinach together until smooth.
2. Add the recommended dosage of the B vitamin complex supplement and blend briefly to mix.

Usage:

Consume this drink in the morning to kickstart your day or before activities that require high energy levels, ensuring optimal absorption and effectiveness.

Benefits:

This energy boost drink aids in the efficient conversion of food into usable energy, reducing fatigue and enhancing mental alertness. Regular intake supports metabolic processes and is beneficial for overall health maintenance, especially in stressful times.

183. Cordyceps Energy Tonic

Description:

Cordyceps mushrooms are prized in traditional Chinese medicine for their ability to increase energy and reduce fatigue by enhancing cellular energy production.

Ingredients:

- Dried cordyceps mushrooms
- 1 cup of hot water
- Honey or lemon to taste (optional)

Preparation Steps:

1. Steep dried cordyceps mushrooms in hot water for at least 10 minutes to make a tea.
2. Strain the mushrooms and add honey or lemon to enhance the flavor if desired.

Usage:

Drink cordyceps tea once daily, preferably in the morning, to harness its energy-boosting properties throughout the day.

Benefits:

Cordyceps tea helps to elevate energy levels and improve stamina by optimizing oxygen utilization and enhancing mitochondrial activity. Regular consumption can lead to increased physical performance and reduced feelings of fatigue, supporting an active and energetic lifestyle.

184. Watermelon Hydration Boost Smoothie

Description:

Watermelon is ideal for hydration and a quick energy boost due to its high water content, natural sugars, and rich electrolyte profile.

Ingredients:

- 2 cups cubed watermelon
- 1/2 cup coconut water (for additional electrolytes)
- A handful of ice
- A sprig of mint for extra freshness (optional)

Preparation Steps:

1. Blend cubed watermelon, coconut water, and ice until smooth.
2. Add mint for a refreshing flavor twist and blend again briefly.

Usage:

Enjoy this smoothie on hot days or after workouts to quickly rehydrate and replenish energy stores with a natural, refreshing drink.

Benefits:

This smoothie offers an excellent way to stay hydrated while providing a natural source of quick-release energy from watermelon's sugars. The addition of coconut water enhances the electrolyte content, supporting optimal hydration and muscle function.

185. Guarana Natural Energy Shot

Description:

Guarana, containing more caffeine than coffee beans, offers a potent energy boost and improves mental focus without the harsh effects often associated with coffee.

Ingredients:

- 1 teaspoon of guarana powder
- 1 cup of cold water
- Honey or a slice of lemon for flavor enhancement (optional)

Preparation Steps:

1. Dissolve the guarana powder in cold water.
2. Add honey or a slice of lemon to taste, if desired, and stir well.

Usage:

Consume this energy shot in the morning or before periods of extended mental or physical activity to maximize alertness and stamina.

Benefits:

Guarana's high caffeine content stimulates the central nervous system, providing rapid energy and heightened focus. Regular use can enhance cognitive performance and endurance, making it ideal for challenging tasks or long days.

186. Citrus Fruit Energy Booster

Description:

Citrus fruits, rich in vitamin C and natural sugars, provide an immediate energy lift and enhanced alertness, making them perfect for a quick and healthy energy boost.

Ingredients:

- Juice of 2 oranges
- Juice of 1 grapefruit
- A dash of lime juice for extra zing

Preparation Steps:

1. Squeeze the juice from the oranges and grapefruit into a glass.
2. Add a dash of lime juice and stir to combine.

Usage:

Drink this citrus blend in the morning or during an afternoon slump to rejuvenate your energy levels and sharpen mental focus.

Benefits:

This citrus mix not only refreshes but also boosts energy levels and mental alertness thanks to the natural sugars and high vitamin C content. It supports immune function and stimulates metabolic processes, aiding in sustained energy throughout the day.

187. Pumpkin Seed Energy Snack

Description:

Pumpkin seeds are a nutrient-dense snack, rich in iron, magnesium, and proteins, making them excellent for sustaining energy levels throughout the day.

Ingredients:

- 1 cup raw pumpkin seeds
- A pinch of sea salt
- Optional: a drizzle of olive oil or sprinkle of paprika for added flavor

Preparation Steps:

1. Roast the pumpkin seeds in a dry skillet over medium heat until they start to pop, about 3-5 minutes.
2. Season with sea salt, and if desired, add a drizzle of olive oil or a sprinkle of paprika for extra flavor.

Usage:

Enjoy a handful of these roasted pumpkin seeds as a mid-morning snack or whenever you need an energy boost during the day.

Benefits:

Pumpkin seeds provide a steady release of energy due to their high protein and magnesium content. The iron in the seeds helps in improving blood oxygen levels, enhancing overall energy and focus. Regular consumption can aid in maintaining balanced energy levels, especially beneficial for active lifestyles.

188. Raw Cacao Energy Booster

Description:

Raw cacao, containing theobromine—a natural

stimulant similar to caffeine—boosts energy and improves mood, offering a wholesome alternative to processed chocolate.

Ingredients:

- 2 tablespoons raw cacao powder
- 1 cup almond milk or any plant-based milk
- 1 tablespoon honey or maple syrup for sweetness (optional)

Preparation Steps:

1. Heat the almond milk in a small saucepan over medium heat until just warm.
2. Whisk in the raw cacao powder until smooth.
3. Sweeten with honey or maple syrup if desired.

Usage:

Drink this warm cacao beverage in the morning or early afternoon to harness its energizing effects and mood-enhancing properties.

Benefits:

Raw cacao boosts energy levels and enhances mood through its natural theobromine content, which stimulates the central nervous system without the jitteriness often associated with caffeine. It's also rich in antioxidants, supporting overall health and well-being.

189. Almond Energy Snack

Description:

Almonds are packed with protein, manganese, copper, and riboflavin, making them an excellent choice for a quick and healthy energy boost.

Ingredients:

- 1 cup raw almonds
- Optional: a pinch of sea salt or a sprinkle of cinnamon for flavor enhancement

Preparation Steps:

1. If desired, toast the almonds lightly in a dry skillet over medium heat for 3-5 minutes until golden and fragrant.
2. Season with a pinch of sea salt or a sprinkle of cinnamon for added flavor.

Usage:

Enjoy a handful of almonds as a mid-morning snack or whenever you need a quick energy lift during the day.

Benefits:

Almonds provide sustained energy due to their high protein content and healthy fats. They also contain essential nutrients like manganese and riboflavin, which are important for energy production and overall metabolic health. Regular consumption can help maintain energy levels and support a healthy lifestyle.

190. Ashwagandha Energy Tonic

Description:

Ashwagandha is known for increasing energy by enhancing the body's resilience to physical and mental stress, making it a powerful adaptogen for improving vitality.

Ingredients:

- 1 teaspoon ashwagandha powder
- 1 cup warm milk or plant-based milk
- Honey or maple syrup to taste (optional)

Preparation Steps:

1. Mix ashwagandha powder into warm milk until fully dissolved.
2. Sweeten with honey or maple syrup if desired.

Usage:

Drink this tonic once daily, ideally in the morning or early afternoon, to maximize its stress-reducing and energy-boosting effects.

Benefits:

Ashwagandha helps increase energy levels and improves stress resistance without the stimulants found in caffeine. Its adaptogenic properties support adrenal health, reducing cortisol levels and enhancing overall energy and mental clarity throughout the day.

191. Yerba Mate Energy Drink

Description:

Yerba Mate is a natural stimulant from South America that enhances alertness and energy through its caffeine content, perfectly aligning with the outlive approach.

Ingredients:

- 1-2 tablespoons of loose Yerba Mate leaves
- 1 cup of hot water (not boiling, to preserve nutrients)

Preparation Steps:

1. Steep the Yerba Mate leaves in hot water for 5-10 minutes.
2. Strain the leaves and serve the brew in a cup.

Usage:

Consume in the morning or early afternoon for a natural energy boost and enhanced mental clarity.

Benefits:

Yerba Mate stimulates energy and focus with a balanced mix of caffeine, theobromine, and theophylline, supporting sustained mental and physical performance.

192. Goji Berry Vitality Snack

Description:

Goji berries, celebrated as a superfood, boost energy and enhance well-being with their high antioxidant content, supporting the longevity-focused approach to health.

Ingredients:

- 1/4 cup dried goji berries
- Optional: Mix with nuts or yogurt for a hearty snack

Preparation Steps:

Enjoy goji berries straight from the package or mixed into yogurt or salads for added texture and nutrition.

Usage:

Snack on goji berries throughout the day to maintain energy levels and support overall vitality.

Benefits:

Rich in antioxidants, goji berries help combat oxidative stress and support cellular health, essential for long-term vitality and energy management.

193. Kombucha Energy Drink

Description:

Kombucha, rich in probiotics, provides a natural energy boost with its trace amounts of caffeine and B vitamins, aligning with a proactive approach to health and vitality.

Usage:

Enjoy kombucha in the morning or early afternoon to capitalize on its energizing effects and support digestive health.

Benefits:

Kombucha not only increases energy levels but also enhances gut health due to its probiotic content, contributing to improved nutrient absorption and overall well-being.

194. Honey Citrus Energizer

Description:

This energizing drink combines the natural sugars of honey with the vitamin C-rich juice of citrus fruits for a quick and healthy energy boost.

Ingredients:

- 2 tablespoons raw honey
- Juice of 1 orange
- Juice of 1 lemon
- 1 cup of water or sparkling water
- Ice cubes (optional)

Preparation Steps:

1. In a pitcher, dissolve honey in freshly squeezed orange and lemon juice.
2. Add water or sparkling water and stir well.
3. Serve chilled with ice cubes if desired.

Usage:

Enjoy this Honey Citrus Energizer in the morning or as a refreshing afternoon pick-me-up to boost energy levels naturally.

Benefits:

This drink not only provides a quick source of energy through honey but also boosts immunity and promotes hydration thanks to the high vitamin C content of citrus fruits.

195. Peppermint Essential Oil Energy Mist

Description:

Peppermint essential oil is known for its ability to enhance physical performance and boost energy when inhaled, making it a quick and effective way to revitalize the mind and body.

Ingredients:

- 10-15 drops of peppermint essential oil
- 1 cup of distilled water
- Small spray bottle

Preparation Steps:

1. Fill the spray bottle with distilled water.
2. Add the peppermint essential oil to the water and shake well to mix.

Usage:

Spray a light mist into the air and inhale deeply to experience an immediate energy boost and enhanced mental clarity. Use before exercise or during a midday slump.

Benefits:

Inhaling peppermint oil stimulates the central nervous system, providing a quick energy surge and improved concentration. It's also known to enhance respiratory functions, making physical activities feel less strenuous.

196. Pomegranate Energy Drink

Description:

Pomegranate juice, rich in antioxidants and natural sugars, enhances blood flow and boosts energy, making it a beneficial drink for maintaining vitality and health.

Ingredients:

- 1 cup of fresh pomegranate juice
- Optional: A splash of lime juice for extra zest

Preparation Steps:

1. Simply pour fresh pomegranate juice into a glass.
2. Add a splash of lime juice for added flavor, if desired.

Usage:

Drink a glass of pomegranate juice in the morning or before physical activity to benefit from its energy-boosting effects.

Benefits:

Pomegranate juice increases energy levels and improves blood circulation, contributing to better oxygen supply to the muscles and brain. Its high antioxidant content also helps protect cells from damage and supports overall health.

197. Sunflower Seed Vitality Snack

Description:

Sunflower seeds, high in vitamin B, help convert food into energy, making them an excellent snack choice for boosting vitality and enhancing metabolic efficiency.

Ingredients:

- 1 cup of raw or roasted sunflower seeds
- Optional: A pinch of sea salt or a sprinkle of cinnamon for flavor enhancement

Preparation Steps:

If desired, lightly roast the sunflower seeds in a dry skillet over medium heat for 3-5 minutes, stirring frequently to prevent burning. Season with sea salt or cinnamon after roasting.

Usage:

Snack on sunflower seeds throughout the day, especially when you need a quick energy lift or a satisfying, nutrient-rich snack.

Benefits:

Sunflower seeds are a powerhouse of energy, thanks to their high content of vitamin B, which aids in energy production. They also provide essential fatty acids, protein, and fiber, supporting overall health and sustained energy levels.

198. Banana Energy Smoothie

Description:

Bananas, with their high potassium and natural sugar content, offer quick energy, making this smoothie ideal for consumption before or during exercise to enhance performance and support the outlive philosophy of sustained health and vitality.

Ingredients:

- 2 ripe bananas
- 1 cup almond milk
- 1 tablespoon honey
- 1/2 teaspoon cinnamon

Preparation Steps:

1. Peel the bananas and place them in a blender.
2. Add almond milk, honey, and cinnamon.
3. Blend until smooth.

Usage:

Drink this banana smoothie about 30 minutes before exercising or during a workout for an immediate energy boost that supports endurance and muscle function.

Benefits:

This smoothie not only provides a quick energy lift from the natural sugars in bananas but also maintains electrolyte balance thanks to potassium, critical for muscle and nerve function. The inclusion of cinnamon adds anti-inflammatory properties, promoting recovery and supporting long-term health and vitality.

SLEEP ENHANCEMENTS

199. Melatonin Sleep Supplement

Description:

Melatonin supplements are effective in regulating the sleep-wake cycle, making them particularly useful for individuals with irregular sleep patterns or those experiencing jet lag, aligning with the outlive approach to enhancing long-term health through improved sleep quality.

Usage:

Take a melatonin supplement according to the dosage instructions on the package, ideally 30-60 minutes before bedtime, especially when adjusting to a new time zone or if struggling to establish a regular sleep pattern.

Benefits:

Melatonin not only facilitates quicker sleep onset but also improves the quality of sleep, ensuring deeper rest and aiding the body's recovery processes. Regular use supports the natural circadian rhythm, essential for overall health and optimal daily functioning.

200. Valerian Root Sleep Aid Tea

Description:

Valerian root is renowned for its sedative properties, which facilitate falling asleep and improving sleep quality, perfectly aligning with the longevity approach to holistic health management.

Ingredients:

- 1 teaspoon dried valerian root
- 1 cup boiling water
- Optional: Honey or lemon to taste

Preparation Steps:

1. Steep the dried valerian root in boiling water for 10-15 minutes.
2. Strain the root and add honey or lemon if desired for flavor.

Usage:

Drink valerian root tea 30-60 minutes before bedtime to enhance relaxation and prepare the body for rest.

Benefits:

Valerian root helps to reduce the time it takes to fall asleep and enhances the overall quality of sleep. Its natural sedative effects promote a deeper, more restorative sleep, supporting the body's natural recovery processes and aiding in long-term health and vitality.

201. Lavender Essential Oil Sleep Mist

Description:

Lavender essential oil, used in aromatherapy, reduces stress and induces relaxation, aiding in faster and deeper sleep, which supports the outlive philosophy of enhancing well-being through natural methods.

Ingredients:

- 10-15 drops of lavender essential oil
- 1 cup of distilled water
- Small spray bottle

Preparation Steps:

1. Fill the spray bottle with distilled water.
2. Add the lavender essential oil to the water and shake well to mix.

Usage:

Spritz the lavender sleep mist around your bedroom and on your pillow before bedtime to create a calming atmosphere that encourages sleep.

Benefits:

Inhaling lavender oil helps lower stress levels and enhances relaxation, promoting a quicker transition to sleep and improving sleep quality. This natural remedy is effective in fostering a restful night, crucial for overall health maintenance and recovery.

202. Chamomile Tea Sleep Enhancer

Description:

Chamomile tea, containing the antioxidant apigenin, binds to brain receptors to promote sleepiness and reduce insomnia, aligning with longevity strategies that emphasize natural sleep aids.

Ingredients:

- 2 tablespoons of dried chamomile flowers
- 1 cup of boiling water
- Optional: Honey or lemon to enhance flavor

Preparation Steps:

1. Steep the dried chamomile flowers in boiling water for 5-10 minutes.
2. Strain the flowers and add honey or lemon if desired.

Usage:

Drink a cup of chamomile tea about 30 minutes before bedtime to help ease into a peaceful sleep.

Benefits:

Chamomile tea not only helps reduce the time it takes to fall asleep but also improves the overall quality of sleep. Regular consumption can help alleviate insomnia, promoting a restful night and supporting the body's natural healing processes.

203. Magnesium Glycinate

Sleep Supplement

Description:

Magnesium Glycinate is a mineral supplement known for its ability to deactivate adrenaline and relax muscles, facilitating easier and more restful sleep, in line with practices that promote sustained health and well-being.

Usage:

Take magnesium glycinate according to the package directions, typically about 30-60 minutes before bedtime, to enhance relaxation and improve sleep quality.

Benefits:

Magnesium glycinate aids in calming the nervous system and relaxing muscle tension, which can help decrease the time it takes to fall asleep and increase sleep duration. Its gentle effect on the body also supports overall sleep quality, essential for optimal health and recovery.

204. Passionflower Tea Sleep Enhancer

Description:

Passionflower tea is known for improving sleep quality by boosting GABA levels in the brain, which helps calm excessive brain activity, aligning with holistic approaches to health for better sleep management.

Ingredients:

- 1 teaspoon of dried passionflower
- 1 cup of boiling water
- Optional: Honey or lemon to taste

Preparation Steps:

1. Steep the dried passionflower in boiling water for 10 minutes.
2. Strain and add honey or lemon if desired for

flavor.

Usage:

Drink passionflower tea about 30-60 minutes before bedtime to promote relaxation and readiness for sleep.

Benefits:

Passionflower tea enhances sleep by increasing GABA levels, which helps reduce anxiety and settle the mind for rest. This natural approach supports deeper and more restorative sleep, crucial for maintaining vitality and health.

205. L-Theanine Sleep Aid Supplement

Description:

L-Theanine, an amino acid found in green tea, promotes relaxation and reduces anxiety, aiding in sleep by facilitating a calmer state of mind.

Usage:

Take L-Theanine as a supplement, following the dosage instructions on the label, ideally in the evening or 30-60 minutes before bedtime to maximize its sleep-promoting effects.

Benefits:

L-Theanine helps to relax the mind without causing drowsiness, making it easier to fall asleep and improving the quality of sleep. It works by moderating levels of certain neurotransmitters, providing a natural way to manage anxiety and promote deeper sleep.

206. Tart Cherry Juice Sleep Enhancer

Description:

Tart cherry juice naturally boosts melatonin levels and contains anthocyanins, compounds that help improve sleep quality by promoting relaxation

and reducing inflammation.

Ingredients:

▫ 1 cup of tart cherry juice

▫ Optional: Water or sparkling water for dilution if the flavor is too strong

Preparation Steps:

1. Serve the tart cherry juice chilled, or dilute with water or sparkling water if preferred.

Usage:

Drink a glass of tart cherry juice an hour before bedtime to benefit from its sleep-enhancing properties.

Benefits:

Consuming tart cherry juice can increase melatonin production, aiding in the regulation of the sleep-wake cycle. The presence of anthocyanins also supports sleep quality by reducing oxidative stress and inflammation, contributing to a more restful night.

207. CBD Oil Sleep Enhancer

Description:

CBD oil, or cannabidiol, helps regulate sleep patterns while reducing anxiety and pain, making it an effective natural remedy for improving sleep quality and managing sleep disturbances.

Usage:

Administer CBD oil sublingually (under the tongue) according to the product's dosage instructions, ideally 30-60 minutes before bedtime to allow its calming effects to take hold.

Benefits:

CBD oil promotes relaxation and eases anxiety, which can significantly improve sleep quality. It also has analgesic properties that can help alleviate pain, further aiding in achieving a restful night without the interruptions often caused by discomfort or stress.

208. Hops Extract Sleep Aid

Description:

Hops extract is traditionally used in herbal medicine for its sedative effects, helping to improve sleep duration and quality by promoting deeper and more restful sleep.

Usage:

Take hops extract in the form of capsules or tinctures, following the recommended dosage on the package. It's best consumed in the evening, about 30-60 minutes before bedtime.

Benefits:

Hops extract has natural sedative properties that facilitate quicker sleep onset and enhance the overall quality of sleep. Its calming effects are especially beneficial for those struggling with insomnia or restless nights, aiding in the natural sleep cycle and supporting restorative rest.

209. Balm Lemon Tea Sleep Enhancer

Description:

Balm Lemon Tea, known for its mild sedative and anti-anxiety properties, acts as a natural remedy conducive to a restful night's sleep, aligning with holistic approaches to health.

Ingredients:

- 1 teaspoon of dried lemon balm leaves
- 1 cup of boiling water
- Optional: Honey or a slice of lemon for flavor

Preparation Steps:

1. Steep the dried lemon balm leaves in boiling water for 5-10 minutes.
2. Strain and add honey or a lemon slice if desired for additional flavor.

Usage:

Drink a cup of Balm Lemon Tea about 30-60 minutes before bedtime to facilitate relaxation and ease into sleep.

Benefits:

Lemon balm tea helps reduce anxiety and promotes calmness, making it easier to fall asleep and improve the quality of sleep. Its gentle sedative effects support a night of deep and restorative sleep, essential for overall well-being.

210. Jasmine Rice Sleep Promoter

Description:

Jasmine rice has a high glycemic index, which can shorten the time it takes to fall asleep when consumed a few hours before bed.

Usage:

Incorporate jasmine rice into your dinner meal, ideally 3-4 hours before bedtime to optimize its sleep-promoting effects.

Benefits:

Eating jasmine rice before bed helps increase the production of sleep-inducing insulin, facilitating quicker sleep onset and a longer, deeper sleep cycle.

211. Kiwi Nighttime Smoothie

Description:

This soothing smoothie uses kiwi, which is rich in serotonin and antioxidants, to support improved sleep onset, duration, and quality.

Ingredients:

- 2 ripe kiwis, peeled and sliced
- 1/2 cup plain yogurt or almond milk
- 1 tablespoon honey
- A few mint leaves for a refreshing touch

Preparation Steps:

1. Blend the kiwi slices, yogurt or almond milk, honey, and mint leaves until smooth.

Usage:

Enjoy this kiwi smoothie about an hour before bedtime to maximize its sleep-enhancing effects.

Benefits:

The combination of kiwi and mint not only calms the mind but also aids the body in preparing for a restful sleep. Kiwi's natural serotonin and antioxidants help regulate sleep cycles and improve overall sleep efficiency.

212. Glycine Sleep Supplement

Description:

Glycine is a supplement known for lowering body temperature at bedtime, signaling to the body that it's time to sleep, thereby improving sleep quality.

Usage:

Consume glycine in powdered form or as capsules, following the package's dosage instructions, approximately 30-60 minutes before going to bed.

Benefits:

Glycine helps facilitate the body's natural cooling process, which is essential for initiating sleep, resulting in faster sleep onset and improved sleep quality throughout the night.

213. Ashwagandha Sleep Aid

Description:

Ashwagandha, an adaptogen, helps manage stress levels, which is crucial for improving sleep quality by promoting relaxation and reducing anxiety.

Usage:

Take ashwagandha in capsule or powder form, as per the recommended dosage on the packaging, about an hour before bedtime to harness its stress-reducing effects.

Benefits:

Regular intake of ashwagandha can significantly reduce stress and anxiety, creating a calmer state conducive to sleep. This helps improve both the ease of falling asleep and the overall quality of rest, supporting better sleep health.

214. Banana Bedtime Smoothie

Description:

Bananas, rich in potassium and magnesium, help relax overstressed muscles and calm the nervous system, making them ideal for a pre-sleep smoothie.

Ingredients:

- 1 ripe banana
- 1 cup almond milk
- A pinch of cinnamon for added flavor

Preparation Steps:

1. Blend the ripe banana with almond milk and cinnamon until smooth.

Usage:

Enjoy this smoothie an hour before bedtime to benefit from the relaxing effects of banana's natural minerals.

Benefits:

The banana in this smoothie aids in muscle relaxation and nervous system calming, facilitating easier sleep onset and improving sleep quality. The addition of magnesium and potassium helps regulate sleep patterns and ensure a restful night.

215. Warm Milk Sleep Aid

Description:

Warm milk contains tryptophan, an amino acid that aids in the production of serotonin and melatonin, crucial for initiating and improving the quality of sleep.

Usage:

Drink a cup of warm milk about 30 minutes before bedtime to maximize its sleep-promoting effects.

Benefits:

The tryptophan in warm milk enhances the production of sleep-regulating hormones, facilitating a smoother transition to sleep and contributing to a deeper, more restful night.

216. Montmorency Cherry Sleep Supplement

Description:

Montmorency cherry supplements are a natural source of melatonin, aiding in reducing sleep disturbances and improving overall sleep quality.

Usage:

Take Montmorency cherry supplements according to the dosage instructions on the package, ideally in the evening or 30-60 minutes before bedtime.

Benefits:

These supplements help regulate the sleep-wake cycle due to their natural melatonin content, promoting quicker sleep onset and fewer night-time awakenings. Regular use supports a more restful and uninterrupted sleep pattern.

217. Essential Oil Sleep Blend

Description:

An essential oil blend of lavender, bergamot, and sandalwood, used in a diffuser, creates a calming atmosphere that is conducive to sleep by promoting relaxation and reducing stress.

Usage:

Add several drops of the essential oil blend to a diffuser filled with water and run it in your bedroom for 30-60 minutes before you go to sleep.

Benefits:

This aromatic blend helps soothe the mind and body, easing you into a peaceful state that encourages deeper sleep. Lavender calms, bergamot reduces stress, and sandalwood brings mental clarity, together enhancing the overall sleep experience.

218. Epsom Salt Relaxation Bath

Description:

An Epsom salt bath utilizes the magnesium in the salts, which is absorbed through the skin, helping to relax the body and prepare it for a restful sleep.

Usage:

Dissolve 1-2 cups of Epsom salt in a warm bath and soak for at least 20 minutes before bedtime.

Benefits:

The magnesium in Epsom salt helps to relax muscles and reduce stress, facilitating easier sleep onset and improving the quality of rest. This natural remedy is especially effective for soothing physical tension and calming the mind before sleep.

219. California Poppy Sleep Aid

Description:

California Poppy extract acts as a mild sedative, improving sleep quality effectively without the risk of dependency.

Usage:

Take California Poppy extract in tincture or capsule form according to the package directions, ideally about 30-60 minutes before bedtime.

Benefits:

California Poppy extract promotes relaxation and aids in achieving deeper, more restful sleep. Its natural sedative properties help to ease the mind and body, making it easier to fall asleep and stay asleep without the concerns associated with synthetic sedatives.

220. Meditation and Breathing Exercises for Sleep

Description:

Techniques such as guided meditation and the 4-7-8 breathing method can significantly improve sleep onset and quality by promoting relaxation and reducing stress.

Usage:

Practice a guided meditation or the 4-7-8 breathing exercise (inhale for 4 seconds, hold for 7 seconds, exhale for 8 seconds) in a quiet, comfortable setting right before bed.

Benefits:

These mindfulness and breathing techniques help calm the mind and prepare the body for sleep, reducing insomnia symptoms and enhancing sleep quality. Regular practice can lead to long-term improvements in sleep health and overall well-being.

221. Nutritional Yeast Evening Smoothie

Description:

This smoothie utilizes nutritional yeast, which is rich in B vitamins, to help regulate sleep patterns and promote a restful night's sleep.

Ingredients:

- 1 banana
- 1 cup spinach
- 1 tablespoon nutritional yeast
- 1 cup almond milk
- 1 tablespoon almond butter

Preparation Steps:

Blend the banana, spinach, nutritional yeast, almond milk, and almond butter together until smooth.

Usage:

Enjoy this smoothie in the evening, about an hour before bedtime, to benefit from the sleep-regulating properties of nutritional yeast.

Benefits:

The B vitamins in nutritional yeast help enhance natural sleep hormones like melatonin, facilitating a smoother transition to sleep. The combination of magnesium from the almond butter and potassium from the banana further supports muscle relaxation and overall sleep quality.

222. White Noise Machine Sleep Solution

Description:

A white noise machine helps drown out disruptive external noises, providing a consistent auditory backdrop that facilitates deeper and more restful sleep.

Usage:

Set up the white noise machine in your bedroom and use it throughout the night to maintain a quiet, soothing sleep environment.

Benefits:

The steady sound of white noise masks environmental noises that can interrupt sleep, such as traffic or loud neighbors. This creates a tranquil atmosphere conducive to sleep, helping you fall asleep faster and stay asleep longer.

223. Saffron Extract Sleep Enhancer

Description:

Saffron extract is recognized for its potential to improve sleep quality and increase sleep time, making it a valuable natural aid for enhancing rest.

Usage:

Take saffron extract in supplement form according to the dosage instructions on the package, ideally about 30-60 minutes before bedtime to maximize its sleep-promoting effects.

Benefits:

Saffron contains antioxidants and bioactive compounds that may help alleviate symptoms of insomnia and improve overall sleep quality. Regular use can contribute to longer sleep duration and a more restful night, supporting the body's recovery processes.

DETOX AND CLEANSING REMEDIES

224. Lemon Water Detox Drink

Description:

Lemon water is a simple and effective way to kickstart the digestive system and liver detoxification each morning, helping to flush out toxins and cleanse the body.

Ingredients:

- 1 fresh lemon
- 1 cup of warm water

Preparation Steps:

1. Squeeze the juice of one lemon into a cup of warm water.

Usage:

Drink lemon water first thing in the morning on an empty stomach to enhance its detoxifying effects.

Benefits:

Starting the day with lemon water stimulates the liver, promoting the elimination of toxins and aiding in digestion. This daily practice can improve overall metabolic health and support the body's natural detoxification processes.

225. Green Tea Detox Enhancer

Description:

Green tea is rich in antioxidants, especially catechins, which enhance liver function and support the body's natural detoxification processes.

Ingredients:

- 1-2 teaspoons of loose green tea leaves or 1 green tea bag
- 1 cup of hot water (not boiling, to preserve antioxidants)

Preparation Steps:

1. Steep the green tea leaves or tea bag in hot water for 2-3 minutes.

Usage:

Drink green tea in the morning or throughout the day to maximize its detoxifying benefits.

Benefits:

Regular consumption of green tea boosts liver health and aids in detoxification, thanks to its high levels of catechins. These antioxidants help reduce oxidative stress and promote overall wellness, enhancing the body's ability to cleanse itself naturally.

226. Activated Charcoal Detox Aid

Description:

Activated charcoal is used occasionally to bind toxins, helping to eliminate them from the body. It's particularly effective in cases of food poisoning or accidental ingestion of other toxins.

Usage:

Take activated charcoal capsules as directed on the package, ideally immediately after exposure to toxins or when experiencing symptoms of food poisoning.

Benefits:

Activated charcoal works by adsorbing toxins in the digestive system, preventing their absorption into the body. This helps to quickly reduce the effects of poisoning and supports the body's detoxification process, aiding in a faster recovery.

227. Dandelion Root Detox Tea

Description:

Dandelion root tea stimulates liver detoxification and promotes digestion by increasing bile flow, making it an excellent herbal remedy for enhancing the body's natural cleansing processes.

Ingredients:

- 1-2 teaspoons of dried dandelion root
- 1 cup of boiling water

Preparation Steps:

1. Steep the dried dandelion root in boiling water for 10-15 minutes.

Usage:

Drink dandelion root tea once or twice a day, preferably before meals to maximize its digestive and detox benefits.

Benefits:

Regular consumption of dandelion root tea supports liver health by stimulating detoxification and enhancing bile production. This not only aids in digestion but also helps in the natural removal of toxins from the body.

228. Milk Thistle Liver Detox Supplement

Description:

Milk thistle supplements protect and promote liver health, the body's primary detoxifying organ, by rebuilding liver cells and removing toxins.

Usage:

Take milk thistle supplements according to the dosage instructions on the package, typically with meals to enhance absorption and efficacy.

Benefits:

Milk thistle supports liver function by protecting it from damage and promoting the regeneration of liver cells. Its silymarin content acts as an antioxidant, aiding in detoxification and overall liver health, crucial for effectively processing and eliminating toxins.

229. Chlorella Detox Supplement

Description:

Chlorella, a type of green algae, effectively binds to heavy metals and aids in their removal from the body, while also boosting the immune system.

Usage:

Consume chlorella in tablet or powder form as recommended on the product packaging, ideally with meals to improve absorption and maximize detox benefits.

Benefits:

Chlorella supports detoxification by binding to heavy metals and facilitating their excretion. It also enhances immune function thanks to its high nutrient content, including vitamins, minerals, and antioxidants, contributing to overall health and resilience.

230. Beetroot Juice Detox Drink

Description:

Beetroot juice is rich in betalains and other compounds that support liver health and promote detoxification, aligning with the longevity approach to enhancing bodily functions naturally.

Ingredients:

- 1-2 fresh beetroots
- 1 cup of water or apple juice for dilution, if desired

Preparation Steps:

1. Juice the fresh beetroots. Dilute with water or apple juice if the flavor is too strong.

Usage:

Drink a glass of beetroot juice daily, preferably in the morning, to support detoxification and liver health.

Benefits:

Beetroot juice enhances the liver's ability to process and remove toxins from the body, thanks to its high content of detoxifying betalains. Regular intake can help maintain optimal liver function and contribute to overall vitality and longevity.

231. Apple Cider Vinegar Detox Tonic

Description:

Apple cider vinegar enhances liver detoxification and improves lymphatic circulation, aiding in the removal of toxins from the body and supporting overall health.

Ingredients:

- 2 tablespoons apple cider vinegar
- 1 tablespoon honey
- 1 cup warm water
- A squeeze of lemon juice

Preparation Steps:

Mix apple cider vinegar, honey, warm water, and lemon juice in a glass until well combined.

Usage:

Drink this detox tonic once daily, preferably in the morning on an empty stomach, to maximize its detoxifying benefits.

Benefits:

This tonic not only supports the liver in its detoxification processes but also aids in improving lymphatic circulation, which is crucial for removing toxins from the body. Regular consumption can help maintain a healthy metabolic rate and support immune function.

232. Turmeric Detox Tea

Description:

Turmeric supports detoxification with its potent anti-inflammatory and antioxidant properties, and it also stimulates bile production, enhancing liver function.

Ingredients:

- 1 teaspoon ground turmeric
- 1 cup boiling water
- A pinch of black pepper (to enhance absorption)
- Honey or lemon to taste

Preparation Steps:

1. Steep ground turmeric and a pinch of black pepper in boiling water for 10 minutes.
2. Strain and add honey or lemon to taste.

Usage:

Drink turmeric detox tea daily, ideally in the morning, to take advantage of its detoxifying and liver-supportive properties.

Benefits:

Turmeric's curcumin boosts liver function by enhancing bile production, crucial for detoxifying the body. Its anti-inflammatory and antioxidant qualities also help protect and heal liver cells from damage caused by toxins.

233. Ginger Detox Tea

Description:

Ginger tea aids in digestion and alleviates nausea while stimulating detoxification by enhancing circulation and promoting sweating.

Ingredients:

- 1-2 inches of fresh ginger root, peeled and sliced
- 1 cup of boiling water
- Honey or lemon to taste

Preparation Steps:

1. Steep the sliced ginger in boiling water for 10-15 minutes.
2. Strain and add honey or lemon to enhance flavor if desired.

Usage:

Drink ginger tea daily, particularly before meals to boost digestion or anytime to aid detoxification.

Benefits:

Regular consumption of ginger tea supports the body's natural detox processes through improved blood circulation and increased sweating, which help remove toxins. Ginger's properties also soothe the stomach and enhance overall digestive health.

234. Cilantro Heavy Metal Detox Smoothie

Description:

Cilantro, known for its ability to bind to heavy metals, facilitates their removal from the body, especially from neurologic tissue.

Ingredients:

- 1 cup fresh cilantro leaves
- 1 banana
- 1/2 cup pineapple chunks
- 1 tablespoon chia seeds
- 1 cup coconut water

Preparation Steps:

1. Combine all ingredients in a blender.
2. Blend until smooth and creamy.

Usage:

Enjoy this detox smoothie once a day to support the body's natural detoxification processes, particularly in removing heavy metals.

Benefits:

The combination of cilantro, banana, pineapple, and coconut water not only provides a refreshing flavor but also supports the body in eliminating heavy metals, aiding in detoxification. Additionally, chia seeds add fiber and omega-3 fatty acids for overall health.

235. Garlic Detox Booster

Description:

Garlic contains sulfur compounds that help activate liver enzymes responsible for expelling toxins from the body, supporting efficient detoxification.

Ingredients:

- 2 cloves of fresh garlic, finely minced
- 1 tablespoon of olive oil
- A squeeze of lemon juice

Preparation Steps:

Combine minced garlic with olive oil and lemon juice to create a simple dressing or marinade.

Usage:

Incorporate this garlic mixture into your daily meals, such as drizzling over salads or vegetables, to enhance flavor and detoxification benefits.

Benefits:

Garlic's sulfur compounds boost liver function by activating enzymes that help clear toxins from the body. Regular consumption can improve overall liver health and aid in the body's natural detox processes.

236. Psyllium Husk Fiber Boost

Description:

Psyllium husk is a fiber supplement that binds to waste material in the digestive tract, aiding in its removal and playing a crucial role in any detox plan.

Usage:

Mix one tablespoon of psyllium husk powder with a glass of water or your favorite beverage. Consume immediately, as it thickens quickly, ideally 30 minutes before meals.

Benefits:

Psyllium husk enhances bowel movements by increasing stool bulk and facilitating the quick and efficient removal of waste and toxins from the digestive tract. Regular use helps maintain digestive health and supports the body's detoxification processes.

237. Burdock Root Detox Tea

Description:

Burdock root, traditionally used as a blood purifier, assists in removing toxins from the bloodstream, enhancing overall detoxification.

Ingredients:

- 1-2 teaspoons of dried burdock root
- 1 cup of boiling water

Preparation Steps:

1. Steep the dried burdock root in boiling water for about 10-15 minutes.
2. Strain the tea into a cup.

Usage:

Drink burdock root tea once or twice a day, preferably before meals, to maximize its blood-purifying properties.

Benefits:

Burdock root tea supports the body's natural detox processes by cleansing the bloodstream and promoting the elimination of toxins through its diuretic properties. This helps enhance overall health and supports the liver and kidneys in their cleansing functions.

238. Watercress Detox Salad

Description:

Watercress acts as a natural diuretic, supports kidney function, and boosts detoxification enzymes in the liver, making it an excellent ingredient for a detoxifying salad.

Ingredients:

- 2 cups fresh watercress
- 1/2 avocado, sliced
- 1 small cucumber, sliced
- 1 tablespoon olive oil
- Juice of 1 lemon
- Salt and pepper to taste

Preparation Steps:

1. Wash and dry the watercress thoroughly.
2. Combine watercress, avocado, and cucumber in a salad bowl.
3. Drizzle with olive oil and lemon juice, then season with salt and pepper.

Usage:

Enjoy this salad as part of your daily meals, particularly beneficial for lunch or as a refreshing side dish to support detoxification.

Benefits:

Watercress enhances the body's detox capabilities by promoting kidney function and increasing liver enzymes that help detoxify the blood. The added ingredients like avocado provide healthy fats and additional nutrients that support overall health and wellness.

239. Seaweed Detox Wrap

Description:

Seaweed is rich in iodine and other minerals that support thyroid function and naturally detoxify the body, making it an excellent ingredient for a nutritious wrap.

Ingredients:

- 2 sheets of nori or any edible seaweed
- 1 cup cooked brown rice
- 1/2 cucumber, julienned
- 1 carrot, julienned
- 1/2 avocado, sliced
- Optional: a splash of soy sauce or a sprinkle of sesame seeds

Preparation Steps:

1. Lay out the seaweed sheets flat.
2. Spread cooked brown rice evenly over each sheet, leaving a small border around the edges.
3. Arrange cucumber, carrot, and avocado slices on top of the rice.
4. If desired, add soy sauce or sesame seeds for extra flavor.

Usage:

Roll up the seaweed sheets tightly, slice into pieces, and enjoy as a detoxifying meal or snack.

Benefits:

Seaweed aids in detoxification through its high iodine content, which supports thyroid health and metabolism. The additional minerals in seaweed also help flush toxins from the body, promoting overall health and vitality.

240. Lymphatic Drainage Massage Guide

Description:

Lymphatic drainage massage is a technique that stimulates the lymph nodes to drain fluids and toxins more effectively from body tissues, enhancing the body's natural detoxification process.

Usage:

Perform lymphatic drainage massage by gently massaging the skin in circular motions towards the heart. Start from the extremities and move inward, focusing on areas with lymph nodes such as the armpits, groin, and neck.

Benefits:

This type of massage helps reduce swelling and detoxifies the body by improving lymph flow. It supports the immune system by facilitating the removal of waste products and toxins from the tissues, thereby promoting overall health and well-being.

241. Sauna Detox Therapy

Description:

Using a sauna promotes sweating, a powerful and natural way for the body to eliminate toxins through the skin, supporting the body's natural detoxification processes.

Usage:

Spend 15-20 minutes in a sauna, followed by a cooling period. Repeat up to three times during a session, and ensure to hydrate adequately before and after to replace lost fluids.

Benefits:

Regular sauna sessions enhance detoxification by significantly increasing sweat production, which helps remove heavy metals and other toxins from the body. This process not only cleanses the skin but also improves cardiovascular health and reduces stress levels.

242. Nettle Tea Detox Drink

Description:

Nettle tea supports kidney function by aiding in the processing and expulsion of waste materials and toxins, enhancing the body's natural detox pathways.

Ingredients:

- 1-2 teaspoons of dried nettle leaves
- 1 cup of boiling water
- Preparation Steps:
- Steep dried nettle leaves in boiling water for 10-15 minutes.
- Strain and serve the tea warm or chilled.

Usage:

Drink nettle tea daily, preferably in the morning or afternoon, to support detoxification efforts and kidney health.

Benefits:

Nettle tea promotes kidney health by facilitating the removal of waste and toxins from the body. Its natural diuretic properties help increase urine production, assisting in cleansing the urinary tract and improving overall urinary and renal function.

243. Pectin-Rich Fruit Smoothie

Description:

Pectin, found in fruits like apples and citrus, supports detoxification by aiding in the removal of heavy metals from the intestines, enhancing the body's natural cleansing processes.

Ingredients:

- 1 large apple, cored and chopped
- Juice of 1 orange
- 1 banana

- □ 1/2 cup of water or apple juice
- □ Optional: 1 tablespoon of lemon juice for added detox benefits

Preparation Steps:

1. Combine the apple, orange juice, banana, and water or apple juice in a blender.
2. Blend until smooth, adding lemon juice if using.

Usage:

Enjoy this smoothie in the morning or as a snack to take advantage of pectin's detoxifying properties.

Benefits:

The pectin in apples and citrus fruits binds to heavy metals and facilitates their elimination from the body, particularly from the digestive tract. Regular consumption can help enhance intestinal health and support overall toxin removal.

244. Green Vegetable Detox Juice

Description:

Juicing green vegetables provides essential nutrients and antioxidants that support detoxification and offer a restorative boost without overburdening the digestive system.

Ingredients:

- □ 2 cups of spinach
- □ 1 cup of kale
- □ 1 green apple, cored and sliced
- □ 1/2 cucumber
- □ 1 celery stalk
- □ Juice of 1/2 lemon

Preparation Steps:

1. Wash all vegetables and the apple thoroughly.
2. Juice the spinach, kale, apple, cucumber, and celery in a juicer.
3. Stir in the lemon juice after juicing for an added detoxifying effect.

Usage:

Drink a glass of green vegetable juice in the morning or between meals to maximize the absorption of nutrients and support the body's natural detox processes.

Benefits:

This juice is rich in chlorophyll, vitamins, and minerals that aid in detoxification and promote liver health. The antioxidants in the greens and apple help neutralize harmful toxins, while the fiber in the ingredients supports healthy digestion and regular elimination.

245. Epsom Salt Detox Bath

Description:

An Epsom salt bath facilitates the removal of toxins through the skin while helping to relieve muscle tension, offering a dual benefit of detoxification and relaxation.

Ingredients:

- □ 2 cups of Epsom salt
- □ Warm bath water

Preparation Steps:

1. Fill your bathtub with warm water.
2. Add 2 cups of Epsom salt to the bathwater and stir until the salts are fully dissolved.

Usage:

Soak in the Epsom salt bath for about 20 minutes to allow the magnesium from the salts to be absorbed through the skin and to maximize the detoxifying effects.

Benefits:

The magnesium in Epsom salt helps to draw out toxins from the body and relaxes the muscles, reducing inflammation and pain. This bath is especially beneficial after physical activities or during times of stress to aid recovery and promote overall well-being.

246. Artichoke Liver Detox Salad

Description:

Artichoke is known for promoting liver function and bile production, crucial for detoxification and fat metabolism, making it an excellent ingredient for a health-enhancing salad.

Ingredients:

- 2-3 cooked artichoke hearts, sliced
- 1 cup arugula
- 1/2 cup cherry tomatoes, halved
- 1/4 cup shaved Parmesan cheese
- Dressing: Olive oil, lemon juice, salt, and pepper

Preparation Steps:

1. Combine arugula, sliced artichoke hearts, cherry tomatoes, and shaved Parmesan in a salad bowl.
2. Whisk together olive oil, lemon juice, salt, and pepper to make the dressing.
3. Drizzle the dressing over the salad and toss gently to combine.

Usage:

Enjoy this artichoke liver detox salad as part of your lunch or dinner to leverage the detox benefits of artichokes.

Benefits:

Artichokes enhance liver health by promoting bile production, which helps eliminate toxins and metabolize fats more efficiently. The fibers and antioxidants in artichokes also support digestive health and overall well-being.

247. Kombucha Detox Beverage

Description:

Kombucha, a fermented tea, contains glucuronic acid which binds to toxins, aiding their rapid removal from the body and supporting detoxification processes.

Ingredients:

- 1 bottle of organic kombucha (preferably plain or ginger flavored for additional detox benefits)

Preparation Steps:

1. Serve the kombucha chilled from the refrigerator. Optionally, you can add a slice of lemon or mint for enhanced flavor.

Usage:

Drink a glass of kombucha daily, preferably in the morning, to capitalize on its detoxifying properties throughout the day.

Benefits:

Kombucha supports liver detoxification through its glucuronic acid content, which helps bind and expel toxins. Additionally, its probiotic properties promote gut health, further enhancing the body's natural detoxification abilities and improving overall digestive function.

248. Schisandra Berry Detox Tea

Description:

Schisandra berries are celebrated for their liver-protective properties and ability to promote the detoxification of harmful substances, enhancing overall liver health and function.

Ingredients:

- 1 teaspoon of dried Schisandra berries
- 1 cup of boiling water

Preparation Steps:

1. Steep dried Schisandra berries in boiling water for about 10-15 minutes.
2. Strain the berries and serve the tea warm.

Usage:

Drink Schisandra berry tea once or twice daily, preferably between meals, to maximize its liver detoxifying effects.

Benefits:

Schisandra berries enhance liver function by promoting the enzymatic processes necessary for detoxifying toxins. Regular consumption can help protect the liver from damage, support its repair mechanisms, and improve overall systemic health through enhanced detoxification.

WEIGHT MANAGEMENT REMEDIES

249. Green Tea Extract Metabolism Booster

Description:

Green tea extract is high in catechins, particularly EGCG (epigallocatechin gallate), which is known to boost metabolism and aid in fat burning, making it a valuable supplement for weight management.

Usage:

Take green tea extract in capsule or liquid form as directed on the product packaging, typically before meals to enhance its metabolic benefits.

Benefits:

EGCG, the active component in green tea extract, increases the rate at which fat is burned in the body, supporting weight loss efforts. It also provides antioxidant benefits that contribute to overall health by reducing inflammation and enhancing cellular repair processes.

250. Apple Cider Vinegar Weight Management Tonic

Description:

Apple cider vinegar helps stabilize blood sugar levels, reduces appetite, and increases feelings of fullness, which can lead to lower calorie intake and aid in weight management.

Ingredients:

- 2 tablespoons apple cider vinegar
- 1 cup of water
- 1 tablespoon honey (optional for sweetness)
- A squeeze of lemon (optional for flavor)

Preparation Steps:

1. Mix apple cider vinegar and water. Add honey and lemon if desired for improved taste.

Usage:

Drink this tonic before meals to maximize the benefits of apple cider vinegar in appetite control and blood sugar stabilization.

Benefits:

Regular consumption of apple cider vinegar can help reduce body weight and body fat mass by promoting satiety and reducing overall calorie intake. Its ability to moderate blood sugar levels also helps prevent spikes and crashes that can lead to overeating.

251. Cayenne Pepper Metabolism Enhancer

Description:

Cayenne pepper contains capsaicin, a compound that boosts metabolism and increases fat burning, making it a potent aid in weight management.

Ingredients:

- 1/4 teaspoon of cayenne pepper

- ☐ 1 cup of warm water
- ☐ Lemon juice from 1/2 lemon (optional for flavor)
- ☐ 1 teaspoon honey (optional for sweetness)

Preparation Steps:

Mix cayenne pepper with warm water. Add lemon juice and honey to enhance flavor if desired.

Usage:

Drink this spicy tonic in the morning or before meals to stimulate your metabolism and enhance fat burning.

Benefits:

Capsaicin in cayenne pepper not only boosts metabolic rate but also promotes increased energy expenditure and fat oxidation, helping to reduce fat stores and manage weight effectively. The addition of lemon and honey can improve the tonic's taste and offer additional health benefits.

252. Konjac Root Fullness Enhancer

Description:

Konjac root, or glucomannan, is a dietary fiber that expands in the stomach, increasing feelings of fullness and reducing overall calorie intake, aligning with longevity practices that emphasize maintaining a healthy weight.

Usage:

Take konjac root supplements with a glass of water about 30 minutes before meals, as per the dosage instructions on the packaging, to maximize its appetite-suppressing effects.

Benefits:

By expanding in the stomach, konjac root helps reduce hunger and prolongs satiety, which can lead to decreased caloric intake and support weight management. This natural approach to controlling appetite contributes to long-term health and wellness, supporting the body's efforts in maintaining an optimal weight as part of a longevity-focused lifestyle.

253. Garcinia Cambogia Weight Control Supplement

Description:

Garcinia Cambogia extract is known for its ability to inhibit the production of new fat in the body and suppress appetite, making it a popular choice for weight management.

Usage:

Take Garcinia Cambogia extract in capsule form as directed on the product packaging, typically before meals to take advantage of its appetite-suppressing and fat-blocking properties.

Benefits:

Garcinia Cambogia contains hydroxycitric acid (HCA), which helps reduce the conversion of carbohydrates into stored fat by inhibiting key enzymes involved in fat production. It also increases serotonin levels, which can help reduce food cravings and decrease overall appetite, supporting effective weight loss and maintenance.

254. Protein Powder Satiety Booster

Description:

Protein powder, whether whey or plant-based, is beneficial for weight management as high-protein diets are linked to greater satiety and reduced overall calorie consumption.

Usage:

Incorporate protein powder into your daily diet by adding it to smoothies, oatmeal, or yogurt. Consume a protein-enhanced meal or snack, particularly before or after workouts, to maximize muscle repair and growth while enhancing satiety.

Benefits:

Consuming high levels of protein helps maintain muscle mass during weight loss, boosts metabolism, and increases feelings of fullness. This leads to a natural reduction in calorie intake and supports sustained weight management, aligning with healthy, long-term dietary habits.

255. Chromium Picolinate Blood Sugar Stabilizer

Description:

Chromium picolinate is a supplement known for its ability to help manage blood sugar levels and may reduce appetite, particularly for carbohydrates, aiding in weight management.

Usage:

Take chromium picolinate according to the package instructions, usually with meals to help stabilize blood sugar levels and reduce cravings throughout the day.

Benefits:

Chromium picolinate enhances the action of insulin, which is crucial for maintaining stable blood sugar levels. By doing so, it helps reduce cravings, especially for carbohydrate-rich foods, and can assist in controlling overall caloric intake. This effect supports sustained weight management and can be particularly beneficial for individuals looking to manage or prevent type 2 diabetes.

256. Forskolin Fat Loss Supplement

Description:

Forskolin, derived from the root of the Coleus forskohlii plant, is believed to enhance fat loss by activating the adenylate cyclase enzyme, which helps break down stored fat and improve metabolism.

Usage:

Take forskolin supplements as directed on the packaging, usually once or twice a day before meals, to maximize its fat-burning effects.

Benefits:

Forskolin stimulates the production of cyclic AMP (cAMP), a molecule that triggers the release of a thyroid hormone that burns fat and calories. This process not only helps reduce body fat but also aids in increasing lean body mass for a more toned physique, making it a valuable addition to weight management and health regimens.

257. White Kidney Bean Carb Blocker

Description:

White kidney bean extract acts as a starch blocker by inhibiting the enzyme responsible for digesting certain carbohydrates, making it effective in preventing the absorption of carbs and aiding in weight management.

Usage:

Take white kidney bean extract supplements just before meals that contain carbohydrates, as directed on the product packaging, to maximize its carb-blocking effects.

Benefits:

By inhibiting the enzyme that digests carbohydrates, white kidney bean extract helps reduce the amount of carbs absorbed by the body, effectively lowering calorie intake from these foods. This can lead to weight loss, especially for those who consume high-carb diets, and supports overall metabolic health.

258. Psyllium Husk Appetite Control Supplement

Description:

Psyllium husk is a form of fiber that aids in appetite control by expanding in the stomach, providing a feeling of fullness which helps reduce overall calorie intake.

Usage:

Mix one tablespoon of psyllium husk with a glass of water and consume immediately before meals. Ensure to drink plenty of water throughout the day to help the fiber function effectively.

Benefits:

Psyllium husk absorbs water and expands in the stomach, which helps prolong satiety and reduce hunger between meals. This effect aids in managing calorie intake and supports weight loss efforts, making it a valuable addition to a diet aimed at achieving and maintaining a healthy weight.

259. Green Coffee Bean Extract Metabolic Enhancer

Description:

Green coffee bean extract contains chlorogenic acid, which can reduce carbohydrate absorption and improve metabolic function, supporting weight loss and overall metabolic health.

Usage:

Take green coffee bean extract supplements as directed on the packaging, ideally before meals to enhance the effects of chlorogenic acid in reducing carb absorption.

Benefits:

Chlorogenic acid in green coffee bean extract helps lower the absorption of carbohydrates and enhances fat metabolism in the liver. These actions can lead to reduced body fat and improved glucose levels, contributing to better weight management and reduced risk of metabolic diseases.

260. Matcha Powder Metabolism Booster

Description:

Matcha powder, derived from ground whole tea leaves, boosts metabolism and increases fat burning more effectively than traditional green tea due to its concentrated form.

Usage:

Incorporate a teaspoon of matcha powder into smoothies, lattes, or even baking recipes. For a direct approach, whisk matcha with hot water to create a traditional matcha tea, consuming it in the morning or before exercise to enhance its metabolic benefits.

Benefits:

Matcha contains high levels of EGCG (epigallocatechin gallate), a catechin known to enhance metabolic rate and increase fat oxidation. Consuming matcha leads to greater energy expenditure and faster fat burning, which can significantly aid in weight management and overall health enhancement.

261. Bitter Orange Weight Management Supplement

Description:

Bitter orange contains synephrine, a compound

that increases fat oxidation and decreases appetite, making it effective for weight management and metabolic enhancement.

Usage:

Take bitter orange supplements as directed on the product packaging, ideally before meals or workouts to maximize the fat-burning and appetite-suppressing effects.

Benefits:

Synephrine in bitter orange stimulates the body's metabolic rate and enhances the breakdown of fat, aiding in weight loss. Additionally, its appetite-suppressing properties help reduce overall calorie intake, which further supports weight management goals.

262. 5-HTP Appetite Control Supplement

Description:

5-HTP (5-Hydroxytryptophan) is a supplement that increases serotonin levels, helping with appetite suppression and reducing cravings, which can contribute to effective weight management.

Usage:

Take 5-HTP supplements as directed on the packaging, typically with meals or as advised by a healthcare provider. It is recommended to start with a low dose and adjust based on effectiveness and tolerance.

Benefits:

By increasing serotonin levels, 5-HTP helps enhance mood and reduce the impulse to eat due to emotional stress. It also suppresses appetite and reduces cravings, particularly for carbohydrates, aiding in a more controlled dietary intake and supporting weight loss efforts.

263. Cinnamon Apple Yogurt Parfait

Description:

This parfait combines cinnamon's blood sugar-regulating benefits with nutritious apples and yogurt, perfect for managing cravings and supporting weight management.

Ingredients:

- 1 cup Greek yogurt
- 1 medium apple, chopped
- 1 tablespoon ground cinnamon
- 1 teaspoon honey
- A handful of granola or nuts

Preparation Steps:

1. Mix Greek yogurt with cinnamon and honey.
2. Layer half the yogurt in a glass.
3. Add a layer of chopped apples.
4. Add a sprinkle of granola or nuts.
5. Repeat layering with remaining yogurt and apples.
6. Top with cinnamon and a drizzle of honey.

Usage:

Enjoy as a breakfast or snack to benefit from the appetite-suppressing effects of cinnamon.

Benefits:

This parfait helps maintain fullness with high-protein yogurt and fiber-rich apples, while cinnamon aids in glucose control and reduces cravings.

264. Flaxseed Nutritional Smoothie

Description:

Flaxseeds are rich in fiber and healthy fats, which

help maintain fullness and satisfaction after meals. This smoothie incorporates flaxseeds to enhance satiety and support a longevity-focused diet.

Ingredients:

- 2 tablespoons ground flaxseeds
- 1 banana
- 1 cup spinach
- 1 cup almond milk
- 1 tablespoon almond butter

Preparation Steps:

1. Blend all ingredients until smooth.

Usage:

Enjoy this flaxseed nutritional smoothie as part of a breakfast or as a filling snack to extend satiety throughout the day.

Benefits:

Flaxseeds provide dietary fiber and omega-3 fatty acids, promoting digestive health and reducing inflammation. This smoothie supports weight management by keeping you full longer and aligns with a diet aimed at long-term health and vitality.

265. Yerba Mate Energy Tea

Description:

Yerba Mate is celebrated for its energizing effects and its ability to increase metabolism and enhance the body's reliance on fat for fuel during exercise, supporting an active and longevity-focused lifestyle.

Ingredients:

- 1-2 tablespoons of loose Yerba Mate leaves
- 1 cup of hot water

Preparation Steps:

1. Steep the Yerba Mate leaves in hot water for 5-10 minutes.
2. Strain the leaves and serve the tea.

Usage:

Drink Yerba Mate tea in the morning or before workouts to boost energy levels and metabolic rate.

Benefits:

Yerba Mate not only provides a natural energy boost but also enhances fat metabolism during physical activity. This makes it a valuable beverage for improving workout efficiency and supporting weight management as part of a healthy lifestyle aimed at maintaining vitality.

266. Spirulina Appetite Control Smoothie

Description:

Spirulina is high in protein and fiber, which can help reduce appetite and prevent overeating, aligning with strategies for maintaining weight and promoting longevity.

Ingredients:

- 1 tablespoon spirulina powder
- 1 banana
- 1 cup fresh spinach
- 1 cup unsweetened almond milk
- A few ice cubes

Preparation Steps:

1. Blend all ingredients until smooth.

Usage:

Enjoy this spirulina smoothie as a filling breakfast or a midday snack to curb hunger and boost nutrient intake.

Benefits:

Spirulina is not only nutrient-dense but also helps in managing hunger, making it easier to control portion sizes and reduce overall calorie intake. Its high protein and fiber content support satiety, essential for weight management and overall health.

267. Hoodia Gordonii Hunger Suppressant Supplement

Description:

Hoodia Gordonii is a succulent plant traditionally used by the indigenous San people of Southern Africa to reduce hunger and thirst during long hunts. It is now utilized in supplements for its appetite-suppressing properties.

Usage:

Take Hoodia Gordonii supplements as directed on the product packaging, typically before meals to help reduce appetite and control caloric intake.

Benefits:

Hoodia Gordonii contains active compounds that may help signal to the brain that you are full, effectively reducing hunger and aiding in weight management. This can be particularly beneficial for those looking to decrease overall calorie consumption as part of a structured diet plan.

268. Chitosan Fat Blocker Supplement

Description:

Chitosan is a dietary fiber derived from shellfish that binds to fat and cholesterol in the stomach, preventing their absorption and supporting weight management.

Usage:

Take Chitosan supplements as directed on the package, usually with water before meals that are high in fat, to maximize its fat-blocking effects.

Benefits:

Chitosan acts as a natural fat binder, reducing the amount of fat and cholesterol absorbed by the body. This helps in managing body weight and may contribute to lower cholesterol levels, aiding in overall cardiovascular health.

269. Coconut Oil Metabolism Boost

Description:

Coconut oil contains medium-chain triglycerides (MCTs) which are metabolized differently than other fats, providing a quick source of energy and aiding in weight loss by increasing metabolic rate.

Usage:

Incorporate coconut oil into your diet by using it as a cooking oil or adding a tablespoon to smoothies or coffee. It can also be used to replace other cooking oils or butters in recipes.

Benefits:

MCTs in coconut oil are quickly absorbed and metabolized by the liver, providing an immediate source of energy that can enhance thermogenesis and fat burning. Regular consumption can help increase energy expenditure, reduce appetite, and support weight management efforts.

270. CLA Supplement for Body Composition

Description:

CLA (Conjugated Linoleic Acid) is a type of fat found in meat and dairy products, noted for its potential to reduce body fat and increase muscle retention, making it a popular supplement for improving body composition.

Usage:

Take CLA supplements as directed on the packaging, typically with meals to help reduce body fat and support muscle growth as part of a balanced diet and exercise regimen.

Benefits:

CLA is believed to enhance the body's metabolic rate, decrease fat deposition, and promote muscle growth. These effects can contribute to a leaner physique and may improve overall health outcomes by reducing fat mass and increasing lean muscle, which is crucial for metabolic health.

271. Dandelion Tea Diuretic Drink

Description:

Dandelion tea acts as a diuretic, increasing the body's urine output which can aid in temporary water weight loss, useful for reducing bloating and enhancing detoxification processes.

Ingredients:

- 1-2 teaspoons of dried dandelion leaves
- 1 cup of boiling water

Preparation Steps:

1. Steep dried dandelion leaves in boiling water for 10-15 minutes.
2. Strain the tea and serve either hot or chilled.

Usage:

Drink dandelion tea once or twice daily, especially in the mornings or whenever experiencing bloating, to maximize its diuretic effects.

Benefits:

Regular consumption of dandelion tea can help manage fluid retention, promote liver function, and support detox processes. Its natural diuretic properties facilitate the removal of excess water and toxins from the body, supporting overall health and well-being.

272. Ginger Metabolism Boosting Tea

Description:

Ginger is known for its ability to enhance calorie burn and reduce feelings of hunger, making it an excellent natural aid for weight management and metabolic enhancement.

Ingredients:

- 1-2 inches of fresh ginger root, peeled and sliced
- 1 cup of boiling water
- Optional: Honey or lemon to taste

Preparation Steps:

1. Steep sliced ginger in boiling water for about 10-15 minutes.
2. Strain the tea into a cup and add honey or lemon if desired for flavor.

Usage:

Drink ginger tea twice daily, preferably before meals, to utilize its metabolism-boosting and appetite-suppressing properties.

Benefits:

Ginger tea helps increase the thermal effect of food, which enhances calorie burning. Additionally, its natural compounds can help suppress appetite, making it easier to manage caloric intake and support weight loss efforts.

273. Mustard Seed Metabolic Enhancer

Description:

Mustard seeds contain compounds that may

increase the metabolic rate, aiding in more efficient calorie burning and contributing to weight management efforts.

Ingredients:

- ☐ 1 teaspoon of mustard seeds
- ☐ 1 tablespoon of water (to activate the seeds)
- ☐ Optional: Mix with vinegar or olive oil for a dressing

Preparation Steps:

1. Crush the mustard seeds with a mortar and pestle.
2. Mix with a small amount of water to release the enzymes.
3. For a salad dressing, blend with vinegar and olive oil.

Usage:

Incorporate activated mustard seeds into meals such as dressings, marinades, or directly sprinkled over food to enhance metabolic effects.

Benefits:

The activation of mustard seeds helps to stimulate the metabolism, potentially increasing the body's calorie-burning capabilities. Regular consumption can assist in maintaining a healthy weight and improving overall metabolic health.

WOMEN'S HEALTH REMEDIES

274. Chasteberry Supplement for Women's Health

Description:

Chasteberry, also known as Vitex, is known for its effectiveness in regulating menstrual cycles and relieving symptoms of premenstrual syndrome (PMS), making it a valuable herbal remedy for women's health.

Usage:

Take Chasteberry supplements as directed on the product packaging, typically once daily in the morning. It's important to continue usage consistently over several months to experience full benefits.

Benefits:

Chasteberry works by influencing hormonal balance, particularly by regulating the levels of prolactin. This helps normalize menstrual cycles and can alleviate common PMS symptoms such as mood swings, breast tenderness, and bloating. Regular use of Chasteberry can significantly improve overall reproductive health and comfort.

275. Evening Primrose Oil Supplement for Women's Health

Description:

Evening Primrose Oil, rich in GLA (gamma-linolenic acid), helps reduce PMS symptoms and menopausal hot flashes, aligning with the longevity approach to enhancing health through natural supplements.

Usage:

Take Evening Primrose Oil capsules as recommended on the product packaging, usually once or twice daily with meals to aid in absorption and effectiveness.

Benefits:

GLA, an essential fatty acid in Evening Primrose Oil, supports hormonal balance, which can alleviate discomfort from PMS and reduce the frequency and severity of hot flashes during menopause. This natural approach to managing women's health issues supports sustained wellness and quality of life through hormonal changes.

276. Black Cohosh Menopause Relief

Description:

Black Cohosh is often used to ease symptoms of menopause, such as hot flashes and night sweats, making it a valued natural remedy for women experiencing menopausal transitions.

Usage:

Take Black Cohosh in capsule or tincture form as directed on the product packaging, typically once or twice daily. It's important to consult with a healthcare provider before starting any new supplement regimen, especially during menopause.

Benefits:

Black Cohosh acts as a natural phytoestrogen, helping to balance hormone levels without the risks associated with traditional hormone replacement therapy. Its use can significantly reduce menopausal symptoms like hot flashes, night sweats, and mood swings, supporting a more comfortable and manageable menopause experience.

277. Red Raspberry Leaf Tea for Women's Health

Description:

Red Raspberry Leaf Tea is traditionally used to strengthen the uterus, improve labor outcomes, and reduce menstrual cramps, making it a staple in women's herbal health practices.

Ingredients:

- 1-2 teaspoons of dried red raspberry leaves
- 1 cup of boiling water

Preparation Steps:

1. Steep the dried red raspberry leaves in boiling water for about 10-15 minutes.

2. Strain the tea and serve hot or chilled, depending on preference.

Usage:

Drink 1-2 cups of red raspberry leaf tea daily, starting in the second trimester of pregnancy to improve labor outcomes, or regularly to ease menstrual cramps and support uterine health.

Benefits:

Red Raspberry Leaf Tea is rich in vitamins and minerals, including magnesium, potassium, iron, and B vitamins, which contribute to its ability to strengthen the uterine walls and improve muscle tone. Regular consumption can lead to easier labor and reduced labor pains, as well as less severe menstrual cramps, supporting overall reproductive health.

278. Dong Quai Hormonal Balance Supplement

Description:

Dong Quai, often referred to as "female ginseng," is renowned for promoting menstrual health and balancing female hormones.

Usage:

Take Dong Quai in capsule, tincture, or tea form as recommended on the product packaging, usually once daily. It is important to consult with a healthcare provider before starting any new supplement, especially for hormonal concerns.

Benefits:

Dong Quai aids in regulating menstrual cycles and alleviating symptoms of hormonal imbalance such as PMS and menopausal symptoms, enhancing overall reproductive health.

279. Calcium Supplement for Bone Health

Description:

Calcium is essential for preventing osteoporosis, particularly critical for women post-menopause, to maintain strong and healthy bones.

Usage:

Take calcium supplements as directed on the packaging, usually with meals to enhance absorption, and in conjunction with vitamin D to optimize bone health.

Benefits:

Calcium is vital for maintaining bone density and strength, reducing the risk of osteoporosis, especially in post-menopausal women where bone loss accelerates.

280. Iron Supplements for Women's Health

Description:

Iron supplements are crucial for women of childbearing age to prevent anemia, particularly important for those experiencing heavy menstrual bleeding.

Usage:

Take iron supplements as directed on the product packaging, ideally with a source of vitamin C to enhance absorption, and avoid taking it with calcium-rich foods or supplements which can inhibit iron absorption.

Benefits:

Iron is essential for producing hemoglobin, which helps carry oxygen in the blood. Adequate iron levels prevent anemia, ensuring energy levels remain stable and overall health is maintained.

281. Soy Isoflavones Hormone Balance Supplement

Description:

Soy isoflavones are phytoestrogens that help balance hormones and are particularly effective in alleviating hot flashes in menopausal women.

Usage:

Take soy isoflavones supplements as directed on the packaging, typically once or twice a day, to help manage menopausal symptoms.

Benefits:

Soy isoflavones mimic estrogen in the body, helping to balance hormonal fluctuations during menopause, which can reduce the frequency and intensity of hot flashes and other related symptoms.

282. Maca Root Hormone Balancing Smoothie

Description:

Maca root enhances libido and balances hormones, making it particularly effective for alleviating menopause-related symptoms such as mood swings.

Ingredients:

- 1 tablespoon maca powder
- 1 banana
- 1 cup almond milk
- 1 tablespoon honey
- A handful of ice cubes

Preparation Steps:

1. Combine maca powder, banana, almond milk, honey, and ice cubes in a blender.
2. Blend until smooth.

Usage:

Enjoy this maca root smoothie in the morning or as a midday snack to benefit from its hormone-balancing effects throughout the day.

Benefits:

Maca root is known for its ability to naturally balance hormone levels, which can enhance mood stability and increase libido, making it a supportive dietary addition for those experiencing hormonal fluctuations during menopause.

283. Folic Acid Pregnancy Support Smoothie

Description:

Folic acid is crucial for pregnancy, supporting fetal development and reducing the risk of birth defects, especially in the brain and spine.

Ingredients:

- 1 cup spinach (rich in natural folate)
- 1 banana (for creaminess and nutrients)
- 1 orange, peeled (for vitamin C and additional folate)
- 1/2 cup fortified almond milk (additional source of folic acid)
- 1 tablespoon chia seeds (for omega-3s and fiber)

Preparation Steps:

1. Blend spinach, banana, orange, almond milk, and chia seeds until smooth.

Usage:

Drink this smoothie daily, particularly in the morning, to ensure an adequate intake of folic acid for pregnant women or those planning to become pregnant.

Benefits:

This smoothie provides a natural source of folic acid, essential for reducing the risk of neural tube defects during fetal development. Regular consumption supports overall pregnancy health and fetal growth.

284. Cranberry UTI Prevention Drink

Description:

Cranberry extract is widely used to prevent urinary tract infections (UTIs), which are more common in women due to its properties that inhibit bacteria from adhering to the urinary tract walls.

Ingredients:

- 1/4 cup pure cranberry juice (unsweetened)
- 3/4 cup water or sparkling water
- A squeeze of lime juice for added flavor

Preparation Steps:

1. Mix the cranberry juice with water or sparkling water.
2. Add a squeeze of lime juice for a refreshing taste.

Usage:

Drink this cranberry mixture daily, especially if you are prone to UTIs, to help prevent infection.

Benefits:

Regular consumption of cranberry juice can help reduce the frequency of UTIs in susceptible individuals by preventing the adhesion of bacteria to the urinary tract, promoting overall urinary health.

285. B Vitamin Booster Smoothie

Description:

This smoothie recipe is designed to naturally boost your intake of B vitamins, supporting energy levels, cellular health, and mood balance throughout the day.

Ingredients:

- 1 cup spinach (rich in B vitamins like folate)

- 1 banana (for vitamin B6 and natural sweetness)
- 1/2 cup Greek yogurt (source of B12 and protein)
- 1/2 cup orange juice (for vitamin C which enhances B vitamin absorption)
- 1 tablespoon sunflower seeds (additional B vitamins and healthy fats)
- 1 tablespoon nutritional yeast (a powerhouse of B-complex vitamins)

Preparation Steps:

1. Combine all ingredients in a blender.
2. Blend until smooth.

Usage:

Enjoy this B Vitamin Booster Smoothie in the morning or as a rejuvenating afternoon snack to maximize the benefits of B vitamins for energy and mood regulation.

Benefits:

This smoothie is packed with natural sources of B vitamins, essential for energy metabolism and neurological functions. Regular consumption can help enhance energy levels, support mental clarity, and maintain healthy skin and muscle tone, contributing to overall well-being.

286. Ashwagandha Mood Stabilizer Smoothie

Description:

Ashwagandha is an adaptogen that supports thyroid function and helps reduce stress and anxiety, making it beneficial for stabilizing mood swings and enhancing overall wellness.

Ingredients:

- 1 tablespoon ashwagandha powder
- 1 banana (for natural sweetness and texture)
- 1 cup almond milk (for a creamy base)
- 1/2 teaspoon cinnamon (for flavor and additional health benefits)
- 1 tablespoon honey (optional, for sweetness)

Preparation Steps:

Blend ashwagandha powder, banana, almond milk, cinnamon, and honey together until smooth.

Usage:

Consume this Ashwagandha Mood Stabilizer Smoothie in the morning or when feeling stressed to benefit from its calming effects.

Benefits:

Ashwagandha enhances the body's resilience to stress and supports thyroid function, which can help regulate energy levels and mood. Regular consumption can lead to reduced anxiety, improved stress management, and overall emotional balance.

287. Flaxseed Hormone Balancing Smoothie

Description:

Flaxseeds are rich in lignans and omega-3 fatty acids, which help balance hormones and support menstrual health, making them an excellent addition to a diet focused on reproductive wellness.

Ingredients:

- 2 tablespoons ground flaxseeds
- 1 cup spinach (for added minerals and vitamins)
- 1 banana (for creaminess and natural sweetness)
- 1 cup unsweetened almond milk (or any plant-based milk of your choice)
- 1 tablespoon chia seeds (for extra omega-3s and fiber)

Preparation Steps:

1. Blend all ingredients until smooth, ensuring the flaxseeds are well incorporated to maximize

nutrient absorption.

Usage:

Drink this hormone-balancing smoothie regularly, especially during the menstrual phase, to alleviate symptoms and promote overall reproductive health.

Benefits:

Flaxseeds' lignans act as phytoestrogens, which can help regulate estrogen levels, while their omega-3 fatty acids reduce inflammation. This combination is beneficial for easing menstrual symptoms like cramping and hormonal fluctuations.

288. Saffron Mood Enhancer Tea

Description:

Saffron is known to alleviate PMS symptoms and acts as a natural antidepressant by increasing serotonin levels, making it a valuable addition to a wellness regimen aimed at improving mental health.

Ingredients:

- A few strands of saffron
- 1 cup of boiling water
- Honey or lemon to taste (optional for flavor enhancement)

Preparation Steps:

1. Steep the saffron strands in boiling water for 5-10 minutes.
2. Add honey or lemon to taste if desired.

Usage:

Drink saffron tea daily, particularly during the days leading up to and during menstruation, to help manage PMS symptoms and enhance mood.

Benefits:

Saffron's unique properties can significantly reduce PMS symptoms such as irritability and depression. It is also effective in uplifting mood by boosting serotonin levels, offering a natural way to enhance emotional well-being.

289. Ginger Menstrual Relief Tea

Description:

Ginger is known to reduce menstrual pain as effectively as NSAIDs, helping to relieve cramps and discomfort during menstruation.

Ingredients:

- 1-2 inches of fresh ginger root, peeled and sliced
- 1 cup of boiling water
- Honey or lemon to taste (optional for flavor enhancement)

Preparation Steps:

1. Steep the sliced ginger in boiling water for 10-15 minutes.
2. Strain the tea and add honey or lemon if desired.

Usage:

Drink ginger tea at the onset of menstrual symptoms or during periods to help alleviate cramps and discomfort.

Benefits:

Ginger's anti-inflammatory and analgesic properties make it an effective natural remedy for menstrual pain. Regular consumption can help decrease the severity of menstrual cramps, offering a comforting and soothing effect during periods.

290. Magnesium-Rich Smoothie for Menstrual

Health

Description:

Magnesium helps reduce menstrual cramps and is effective in decreasing the severity of PMS symptoms, supporting overall menstrual health.

Ingredients:

- 1 banana (a good source of magnesium)
- 1/2 cup spinach (rich in magnesium and iron)
- 1 tablespoon pumpkin seeds (high in magnesium)
- 1 cup almond milk (for added calcium and a creamy texture)
- 1 tablespoon cocoa powder (optional for a chocolatey flavor and extra magnesium)

Preparation Steps:

1. Blend all ingredients until smooth.

Usage:

Consume this magnesium-rich smoothie regularly, especially during the week leading up to and during your menstrual period, to help alleviate cramps and reduce PMS symptoms.

Benefits:

Magnesium plays a crucial role in muscle relaxation and nerve function, which can help mitigate menstrual cramps and reduce the overall impact of PMS. This smoothie provides a natural and tasty way to increase your magnesium intake, promoting better menstrual health and comfort.

291. Turmeric Relief Smoothie

Description:

Turmeric is celebrated for its anti-inflammatory properties, which can help alleviate menstrual pain and hormonal acne, making it a valuable addition to a wellness-focused diet.

Ingredients:

- 1 teaspoon of turmeric powder
- 1 cup of coconut milk
- 1 banana (to add creaminess and natural sweetness)
- 1/2 teaspoon of ground cinnamon (for added flavor and anti-inflammatory benefits)
- A pinch of black pepper (to enhance turmeric absorption)
- 1 tablespoon of honey (optional, for sweetness)

Preparation Steps:

1. Blend all ingredients until smooth.

Usage:

Enjoy this turmeric smoothie during menstrual periods or whenever experiencing hormonal acne flare-ups to benefit from its anti-inflammatory effects.

Benefits:

Turmeric contains curcumin, a compound known for its potent anti-inflammatory and antioxidant properties. Regular consumption can help reduce menstrual pain and the occurrence of hormonal acne by controlling inflammation and supporting overall skin health.

292. St. John's Wort Mood Stabilizer Tea

Description:

St. John's Wort is widely recognized for its effectiveness in treating mood disorders and can be particularly helpful in managing mood swings associated with menstrual cycles or menopause.

Ingredients:

- 1-2 teaspoons of dried St. John's Wort
- 1 cup of boiling water
- Honey or lemon to taste (optional for flavor

enhancement)

Preparation Steps:

1. Steep dried St. John's Wort in boiling water for about 10 minutes.

2. Strain the tea and add honey or lemon if desired for better taste.

Usage:

Drink St. John's Wort tea once or twice daily, especially during times when mood swings are prevalent, such as before or during menstruation and throughout menopause.

Benefits:

St. John's Wort helps stabilize mood by influencing neurotransmitters in the brain. Its natural antidepressant properties can alleviate symptoms of depression and mood swings, providing relief during hormonal fluctuations associated with menstrual cycles and menopause.

293. Peppermint Oil Menstrual Pain Relief

Description:

Peppermint oil is effective in reducing menstrual pain when applied topically on the abdomen, offering a soothing and natural remedy for cramps.

Ingredients:

- A few drops of peppermint essential oil
- 1 tablespoon of carrier oil (such as coconut oil or almond oil)

Preparation Steps:

1. Mix a few drops of peppermint essential oil with the carrier oil to dilute.

Usage:

Gently massage the oil mixture onto the abdomen in circular motions. Apply as needed during menstrual periods to help alleviate pain and discomfort.

Benefits:

Peppermint oil has natural analgesic and antispasmodic properties, which help to relax the muscles and reduce pain. The cooling sensation also provides immediate relief, making it an effective and natural option for managing menstrual cramps.

294. Motherwort Reproductive Health Tea

Description:

Motherwort is traditionally used to improve reproductive health, reduce anxiety, and manage heart symptoms associated with menopause, making it a versatile herb for women's health.

Ingredients:

- 1-2 teaspoons dried motherwort
- 1 cup boiling water
- Honey or lemon to taste (optional for flavor)

Preparation Steps:

1. Steep the dried motherwort in boiling water for 10-15 minutes.

2. Strain the tea and add honey or lemon if desired.

Usage:

Drink motherwort tea once or twice daily to support reproductive health, reduce anxiety, and manage menopause-related heart symptoms.

Benefits:

Motherwort helps regulate menstrual cycles, alleviate anxiety, and support heart health, particularly beneficial during menopause. Its calming properties promote overall well-being and reproductive health.

295. Licorice Root

Hormonal Balance Tea

Description:

Licorice root helps modulate estrogen and progesterone balances, making it beneficial for hormonal regulation and supporting women's health.

Ingredients:

- 1 teaspoon dried licorice root
- 1 cup boiling water
- Honey or lemon to taste (optional for flavor)

Preparation Steps:

1. Steep the dried licorice root in boiling water for 10-15 minutes.
2. Strain the tea and add honey or lemon if desired.

Usage:

Drink licorice root tea once daily to help balance hormones and support overall reproductive health.

Benefits:

Licorice root aids in regulating estrogen and progesterone levels, helping to alleviate symptoms related to hormonal imbalances. Regular consumption can support menstrual health, reduce PMS symptoms, and promote overall hormonal well-being.

296. Aloe Vera Digestive Health Juice

Description:

Aloe Vera is known for its soothing properties when applied topically and can also be taken orally to support digestive health, which is often compromised during hormonal changes.

Ingredients:

- 1/4 cup fresh aloe vera gel (from the inner leaf)
- 1 cup water or fresh juice (such as orange or apple juice)
- 1 tablespoon honey (optional for sweetness)

Preparation Steps:

1. Scoop the fresh aloe vera gel from the inner leaf.
2. Blend the aloe vera gel with water or juice until smooth.
3. Add honey if desired for sweetness.

Usage:

Drink this Aloe Vera juice once daily, preferably in the morning, to help soothe and support digestive health.

Benefits:

Aloe Vera aids in digestion and helps reduce inflammation in the gut, promoting overall digestive health. Regular intake can alleviate symptoms such as bloating and discomfort, which may be exacerbated by hormonal changes. Additionally, Aloe Vera's soothing properties can help maintain a healthy digestive system.

297. Probiotic-Rich Yogurt Parfait

Description:

Probiotics support gut health, which is crucial for proper hormone synthesis and detoxification, making them an essential part of a balanced diet.

Ingredients:

- 1 cup plain Greek yogurt (rich in probiotics)
- 1/2 cup fresh berries (such as blueberries, strawberries, or raspberries)
- 1 tablespoon honey (optional for sweetness)
- 1 tablespoon chia seeds (for added fiber and omega-3s)

◻ 1/4 cup granola (for crunch and additional fiber)

Preparation Steps:

1. Layer the Greek yogurt in a bowl or glass.

2. Add fresh berries on top of the yogurt.

3. Drizzle with honey if desired.

4. Sprinkle chia seeds and granola over the berries.

Usage:

Enjoy this probiotic-rich yogurt parfait as a breakfast or a healthy snack to support gut health and hormone balance.

Benefits:

Probiotics in Greek yogurt help maintain a healthy gut microbiome, essential for efficient hormone synthesis and detoxification. The added berries, chia seeds, and granola provide fiber, antioxidants, and omega-3s, enhancing overall digestive and hormonal health.

298. Tea Tree Oil Acne Treatment

Description:

Tea Tree Oil is renowned for its antibacterial properties, making it effective in treating acne, particularly during hormonal changes.

Ingredients:

◻ A few drops of tea tree essential oil

◻ 1 tablespoon of carrier oil (such as jojoba oil or coconut oil)

Preparation Steps:

1. Mix a few drops of tea tree essential oil with the carrier oil to dilute.

Usage:

Apply the mixture to clean, dry skin, focusing on acne-prone areas. Use a cotton swab to dab the oil blend onto blemishes. Leave on overnight or for several hours before rinsing off with warm water.

Benefits:

Tea Tree Oil helps to reduce acne by killing bacteria and reducing inflammation. Its natural antiseptic properties make it an effective treatment for breakouts, particularly those that occur due to hormonal fluctuations. Regular application can lead to clearer, healthier skin.

MEN'S HEALTH REMEDIES

299. Saw Palmetto Prostate Health Supplement

Description:

Saw Palmetto extract is commonly used to support prostate health and treat symptoms of benign prostatic hyperplasia (BPH), making it a valuable remedy for men's health.

Usage:

Take Saw Palmetto extract supplements as directed on the product packaging, typically once or twice daily with meals.

Benefits:

Saw Palmetto helps reduce symptoms of BPH such as frequent urination and difficulty in starting urination. It supports overall prostate health and may improve urinary function, contributing to better quality of life for men experiencing prostate issues.

300. Lycopene-Rich Tomato Salad

Description:

Lycopene, found in tomatoes, helps reduce the risk of prostate cancer and supports overall prostate health, making it an essential nutrient for men.

Ingredients:

- 2 large tomatoes, chopped
- 1/2 red onion, thinly sliced
- 1 cucumber, chopped
- 1/4 cup fresh basil leaves, torn
- 2 tablespoons olive oil
- 1 tablespoon balsamic vinegar
- Salt and pepper to taste

Preparation Steps:

1. Combine the chopped tomatoes, red onion, cucumber, and basil leaves in a large bowl.
2. Drizzle with olive oil and balsamic vinegar.
3. Season with salt and pepper to taste.
4. Toss gently to combine.

Usage:

Enjoy this lycopene-rich tomato salad as a side dish or a light meal to support prostate health.

Benefits:

Tomatoes are an excellent source of lycopene, a powerful antioxidant that helps reduce the risk of prostate cancer and supports overall prostate health. Regular consumption of lycopene-rich foods can contribute to better prostate function and reduce the risk of prostate-related issues.

301. Omega-3 Rich Salmon Salad

Description:

Omega-3 fatty acids are crucial for heart health, reducing inflammation, and supporting cognitive function, making them essential for men's overall health.

Ingredients:

- 1 fillet of cooked salmon (rich in omega-3s)
- 4 cups mixed greens (spinach, arugula, kale)
- 1/2 avocado, sliced
- 1/4 cup walnuts (additional omega-3 source)
- 1/2 red bell pepper, sliced
- 1 tablespoon chia seeds (optional for extra omega-3s)
- 2 tablespoons olive oil
- 1 tablespoon lemon juice
- Salt and pepper to taste

Preparation Steps:

1. Place mixed greens in a large bowl.
2. Top with cooked salmon, avocado, walnuts, red bell pepper, and chia seeds.
3. Drizzle with olive oil and lemon juice.
4. Season with salt and pepper.
5. Toss gently to combine.

Usage:

Enjoy this Omega-3 rich salmon salad for lunch or dinner to support heart health, reduce inflammation, and enhance cognitive function.

Benefits:

Salmon and walnuts are excellent sources of omega-3 fatty acids, which are vital for maintaining cardiovascular health, reducing chronic inflammation, and supporting brain health. Regular consumption of omega-3 rich foods can help protect against heart disease and cognitive decline, contributing to overall well-being.

302. Zinc-Rich Pumpkin Seed and Quinoa Salad

Description:

This salad combines zinc-rich ingredients like pumpkin seeds and quinoa to support testosterone production and improve sperm quality.

Ingredients:

- 1 cup cooked quinoa
- 1/4 cup pumpkin seeds
- 1/2 cup chickpeas, drained and rinsed
- 1/2 avocado, diced
- 1/2 cup cherry tomatoes, halved
- 2 tablespoons chopped parsley
- 2 tablespoons olive oil
- 1 tablespoon lemon juice
- Salt and pepper to taste

Preparation Steps:

1. Cook quinoa according to package instructions and let it cool.
2. In a large bowl, combine cooked quinoa, pumpkin seeds, chickpeas, avocado, cherry tomatoes, and parsley.
3. Drizzle with olive oil and lemon juice.
4. Season with salt and pepper.
5. Toss gently to combine.

Usage:

Enjoy this salad as a nutritious lunch or dinner to boost your zinc intake and support overall men's health.

Benefits:

Pumpkin seeds and quinoa are excellent sources of zinc, essential for testosterone production and enhancing sperm quality, contributing to improved fertility and reproductive health.

303. Pumpkin Seed and Spinach Smoothie

Description:

Pumpkin seeds are rich in zinc and magnesium, which are beneficial for prostate health and testosterone levels, making this smoothie a powerful addition to men's health routines.

Ingredients:

- 1/4 cup pumpkin seeds
- 1 cup fresh spinach
- 1 banana
- 1 cup almond milk
- 1 tablespoon honey (optional for sweetness)
- A handful of ice cubes

Preparation Steps:

1. Blend pumpkin seeds, spinach, banana, almond milk, honey, and ice cubes until smooth.

Usage:

Drink this pumpkin seed and spinach smoothie as a nutritious breakfast or post-workout snack to boost zinc and magnesium intake.

Benefits:

Pumpkin seeds provide zinc and magnesium, essential for maintaining prostate health and supporting healthy testosterone levels, contributing to overall men's health and well-being.

304. Fenugreek Energy Booster Smoothie

Description:

Fenugreek has been shown to boost testosterone levels and enhance libido, making it an excellent addition to a smoothie for men's health.

Ingredients:

- 1 teaspoon fenugreek powder
- 1 banana
- 1 cup unsweetened almond milk
- 1 tablespoon almond butter
- 1/2 teaspoon cinnamon
- 1 tablespoon honey (optional for sweetness)

- A handful of ice cubes

Preparation Steps:

1. Blend fenugreek powder, banana, almond milk, almond butter, cinnamon, honey, and ice cubes until smooth.

Usage:

Enjoy this fenugreek energy booster smoothie in the morning or as a midday snack to support testosterone levels and enhance libido.

Benefits:

Fenugreek is known to naturally boost testosterone and improve libido. Combined with other nutritious ingredients, this smoothie supports overall men's health and energy levels.

305. Ginseng Libido Boosting Smoothie

Description:

Ginseng is known for enhancing erectile function and improving sexual performance, making it an ideal ingredient for a men's health smoothie.

Ingredients:

- 1 teaspoon ginseng powder or extract
- 1 banana
- 1 cup almond milk
- 1 tablespoon honey
- 1/2 teaspoon vanilla extract
- A handful of ice cubes

Preparation Steps:

1. Blend ginseng powder, banana, almond milk, honey, vanilla extract, and ice cubes until smooth.

Usage:

Drink this ginseng smoothie in the morning or before an evening date to boost sexual performance and energy levels.

Benefits:

Ginseng helps enhance erectile function and improves sexual performance, while the other ingredients provide essential nutrients and energy, supporting overall men's health and vitality.

306. Garlic and Spinach Pesto Pasta

Description:

Garlic helps reduce blood pressure and cholesterol, crucial for cardiovascular health, which is often a concern for men.

Ingredients:

- 2 cups fresh spinach
- 3 cloves garlic
- 1/4 cup olive oil
- 1/4 cup walnuts (optional for added texture and omega-3s)
- 1/4 cup grated Parmesan cheese
- 1 tablespoon lemon juice
- Salt and pepper to taste
- 8 ounces whole wheat pasta

Preparation Steps:

1. Cook the pasta according to package instructions and drain.

2. In a food processor, combine spinach, garlic, olive oil, walnuts, Parmesan cheese, lemon juice, salt, and pepper.

3. Blend until smooth.

4. Toss the cooked pasta with the spinach-garlic pesto until well coated.

Usage:

Enjoy this garlic and spinach pesto pasta as a heart-healthy lunch or dinner to benefit from the cardiovascular benefits of garlic.

Benefits:

Garlic helps lower blood pressure and cholesterol levels, supporting cardiovascular health. Combined with nutrient-rich spinach and healthy fats from olive oil, this dish promotes overall well-being and heart health.

307. Vitamin D Boosting Smoothie

Description:

Vitamin D is linked to testosterone production and overall health, and many men are deficient in this crucial nutrient. This smoothie is designed to help boost vitamin D levels.

Ingredients:

- 1 cup fortified orange juice (high in vitamin D)
- 1/2 cup Greek yogurt (rich in vitamin D and calcium)
- 1 banana
- 1 tablespoon chia seeds (for added nutrients)
- 1/2 teaspoon vanilla extract
- A handful of ice cubes

Preparation Steps:

Blend the fortified orange juice, Greek yogurt, banana, chia seeds, vanilla extract, and ice cubes until smooth.

Usage:

Enjoy this vitamin D boosting smoothie in the morning to start your day with a nutrient-packed drink.

Benefits:

Fortified orange juice and Greek yogurt provide a good dose of vitamin D, essential for testosterone production and overall health. This smoothie supports bone health, immune function, and

hormonal balance.

308. Horny Goat Weed Libido Enhancing Smoothie

Description:

Horny Goat Weed is a traditional Chinese medicinal herb used to treat erectile dysfunction and boost libido, making it a valuable ingredient for men's health.

Ingredients:

- 1 teaspoon Horny Goat Weed powder or extract
- 1 banana
- 1 cup almond milk
- 1 tablespoon honey
- 1 tablespoon cocoa powder (optional for added flavor)
- A handful of ice cubes

Preparation Steps:

1. Blend Horny Goat Weed powder, banana, almond milk, honey, cocoa powder, and ice cubes until smooth.

Usage:

Drink this libido-enhancing smoothie in the morning or before an intimate evening to support sexual performance and desire.

Benefits:

Horny Goat Weed helps improve erectile function and boost libido, while the other ingredients provide essential nutrients and energy. Regular consumption can support overall sexual health and vitality.

309. Tribulus Terrestris Testosterone Boosting

Smoothie

Description:

Tribulus Terrestris is popular in traditional medicine for raising testosterone levels and enhancing sexual function, making it an ideal ingredient for a men's health smoothie.

Ingredients:

- 1 teaspoon Tribulus Terrestris powder or extract
- 1 cup unsweetened almond milk
- 1 banana
- 1 tablespoon almond butter
- 1 tablespoon honey (optional for sweetness)
- A handful of ice cubes

Preparation Steps:

1. Blend Tribulus Terrestris powder, almond milk, banana, almond butter, honey, and ice cubes until smooth.

Usage:

Consume this testosterone-boosting smoothie in the morning or before a workout to support testosterone levels and sexual health.

Benefits:

Tribulus Terrestris helps increase testosterone levels and enhance sexual function. Combined with nutrient-dense ingredients, this smoothie supports overall men's health, energy, and vitality.

310. Ashwagandha Vitality Smoothie

Description:

Ashwagandha, an adaptogen, increases stamina, reduces stress, and improves overall vitality, making it a powerful addition to a health-boosting smoothie.

Ingredients:

- 1 teaspoon ashwagandha powder
- 1 banana
- 1 cup unsweetened almond milk
- 1 tablespoon almond butter
- 1/2 teaspoon cinnamon
- 1 tablespoon honey (optional for sweetness)
- A handful of ice cubes

Preparation Steps:

1. Blend ashwagandha powder, banana, almond milk, almond butter, cinnamon, honey, and ice cubes until smooth.

Usage:

Drink this ashwagandha vitality smoothie in the morning or as a mid-afternoon pick-me-up to boost energy levels and reduce stress.

Benefits:

Ashwagandha helps enhance stamina, reduce stress, and improve overall vitality. Combined with other nutritious ingredients, this smoothie supports men's health, energy, and well-being.

311. Maca Root Energy Smoothie

Description:

Maca root enhances energy, stamina, and sexual health, making it a valuable ingredient for a men's health smoothie.

Ingredients:

- 1 tablespoon maca powder
- 1 banana
- 1 cup unsweetened almond milk
- 1 tablespoon peanut butter
- 1 teaspoon honey (optional for sweetness)
- A handful of ice cubes

Preparation Steps:

1. Blend maca powder, banana, almond milk, peanut butter, honey, and ice cubes until smooth.

Usage:

Enjoy this maca root energy smoothie in the morning or before a workout to boost energy levels and support sexual health.

Benefits:

Maca root is known for enhancing energy, stamina, and sexual health. Combined with nutrient-rich ingredients, this smoothie supports overall men's vitality and well-being.

312. Brazil Nut Hormone Balance Smoothie

Description:

Brazil nuts are high in selenium, which is important for prostate health and overall hormonal balance, making them an excellent addition to a men's health smoothie.

Ingredients:

- 2-3 Brazil nuts
- 1 banana
- 1 cup unsweetened almond milk
- 1 tablespoon chia seeds
- 1 tablespoon honey (optional for sweetness)
- A handful of ice cubes

Preparation Steps:

1. Blend Brazil nuts, banana, almond milk, chia seeds, honey, and ice cubes until smooth.

Usage:

Enjoy this Brazil nut hormone balance smoothie in the morning or as a snack to support prostate health and hormonal balance.

Benefits:

Brazil nuts provide a rich source of selenium, essential for maintaining prostate health and supporting overall hormonal balance. This smoothie combines nutrient-dense ingredients to enhance men's health and vitality.

313. Green Tea Antioxidant Smoothie

Description:

Green tea is rich in antioxidants, supporting cellular health and providing protective benefits against prostate cancer, making it a powerful addition to a men's health smoothie.

Ingredients:

- 1 cup brewed green tea, cooled
- 1 banana
- 1/2 cup spinach
- 1/2 cup Greek yogurt
- 1 tablespoon honey (optional for sweetness)
- A handful of ice cubes

Preparation Steps:

1. Brew green tea and let it cool.
2. Blend the cooled green tea, banana, spinach, Greek yogurt, honey, and ice cubes until smooth.

Usage:

Enjoy this green tea antioxidant smoothie in the morning or as an afternoon pick-me-up to boost your antioxidant intake and support overall health.

Benefits:

Green tea is rich in antioxidants that support cellular health and provide protective benefits against prostate cancer. This smoothie combines green tea with nutrient-dense ingredients to enhance men's health and vitality.

314. Pomegranate Heart Health Smoothie

Description:

Pomegranate juice is rich in antioxidants, which can improve heart health and potentially slow the progression of prostate cancer, making it an excellent ingredient for a men's health smoothie.

Ingredients:

- 1 cup pomegranate juice
- 1/2 cup Greek yogurt
- 1 banana
- 1/2 cup frozen berries (such as blueberries or strawberries)
- 1 tablespoon honey (optional for sweetness)
- A handful of ice cubes

Preparation Steps:

1. Blend pomegranate juice, Greek yogurt, banana, frozen berries, honey, and ice cubes until smooth.

Usage:

Enjoy this pomegranate heart health smoothie in the morning or as a refreshing snack to support cardiovascular and prostate health.

Benefits:

Pomegranate juice is rich in antioxidants that can improve heart health and potentially slow prostate cancer progression. This smoothie combines pomegranate juice with other nutritious ingredients to enhance men's overall health and well-being.

315. Oyster Zinc Boost Recipe

Description:

Oysters are high in zinc, which is crucial for men's fertility and sexual health, making them a nutritious addition to a diet focused on men's health.

Ingredients:

- 12 fresh oysters
- 1 lemon, cut into wedges
- Hot sauce (optional)
- Crushed ice for serving

Preparation Steps:

1. Shuck the oysters, carefully opening the shells and keeping the oysters intact.
2. Arrange the oysters on a bed of crushed ice on a serving platter.
3. Serve with lemon wedges and hot sauce on the side.

Usage:

Enjoy oysters as an appetizer or a nutritious snack to boost zinc intake and support fertility and sexual health.

Benefits:

Oysters are an excellent source of zinc, essential for maintaining healthy testosterone levels and supporting sperm production. Regular consumption can enhance fertility and improve sexual health.

316. Nettle Root Prostate Health Tea

Description:

Nettle root supports prostate health and helps manage symptoms associated with an enlarged prostate, making it a beneficial herbal remedy for men.

Ingredients:

- 1 teaspoon dried nettle root
- 1 cup boiling water
- Honey or lemon to taste (optional for flavor)

Preparation Steps:

1. Steep the dried nettle root in boiling water for 10-15 minutes.
2. Strain the tea and add honey or lemon if desired.

Usage:

Drink nettle root tea once or twice daily to support prostate health and manage symptoms of an enlarged prostate.

Benefits:

Nettle root helps reduce symptoms of an enlarged prostate, such as frequent urination, and supports overall prostate health. Regular consumption can improve urinary function and enhance quality of life.

317. Flaxseed Prostate Health Smoothie

Description:

Flaxseeds contain omega-3 fatty acids and lignans that may help prevent prostate cancer, making them a valuable ingredient for a men's health smoothie.

Ingredients:

- 2 tablespoons ground flaxseeds
- 1 banana
- 1 cup almond milk
- 1/2 cup frozen blueberries
- 1 tablespoon honey (optional for sweetness)
- A handful of ice cubes

Preparation Steps:

1. Blend ground flaxseeds, banana, almond milk, frozen blueberries, honey, and ice cubes until smooth.

Usage:

Enjoy this flaxseed prostate health smoothie in the morning or as a snack to support prostate health and overall well-being.

Benefits:

Flaxseeds provide omega-3 fatty acids and lignans, which may help prevent prostate cancer. This smoothie combines flaxseeds with other nutrient-rich ingredients to support men's health and vitality.

318. Cordyceps Energy Boost Smoothie

Description:

Cordyceps boosts energy levels and improves physical performance, with potential benefits for sexual health, making it an excellent addition to a men's health smoothie.

Ingredients:

- 1 teaspoon cordyceps powder
- 1 banana
- 1 cup unsweetened almond milk
- 1 tablespoon almond butter
- 1 tablespoon honey (optional for sweetness)
- A handful of ice cubes

Preparation Steps:

1. Blend cordyceps powder, banana, almond milk, almond butter, honey, and ice cubes until smooth.

Usage:

Enjoy this cordyceps energy boost smoothie in the morning or before a workout to enhance energy levels and support physical performance.

Benefits:

Cordyceps enhances energy and physical performance, while also potentially improving sexual health. This smoothie combines cordyceps with other nutritious ingredients to support overall men's health and vitality.

319. Boron-Rich Smoothie for Testosterone Boost

Description:

Boron is a trace mineral that can naturally increase testosterone levels, making it beneficial for men's hormonal health.

Ingredients:

- 1/2 avocado (rich in boron)
- 1 banana
- 1 cup unsweetened almond milk
- 1 tablespoon almond butter
- 1 tablespoon honey (optional for sweetness)
- A handful of ice cubes

Preparation Steps:

1. Blend avocado, banana, almond milk, almond butter, honey, and ice cubes until smooth.

Usage:

Enjoy this boron-rich smoothie in the morning or as a midday snack to support testosterone levels and overall health.

Benefits:

Avocado and almond butter are good sources of boron, which can help increase testosterone levels naturally. This smoothie combines these ingredients with other nutrients to support men's health and vitality.

320. Curcumin Anti-Inflammatory Smoothie

Description:

Curcumin, found in turmeric, has anti-inflammatory properties that can help prevent prostate cancer and support overall cellular health.

Ingredients:

- 1 teaspoon turmeric powder (curcumin)
- 1 banana
- 1 cup unsweetened almond milk
- 1/2 teaspoon black pepper (enhances curcumin absorption)
- 1 tablespoon honey (optional for sweetness)
- A handful of ice cubes

Preparation Steps:

1. Blend turmeric powder, banana, almond milk, black pepper, honey, and ice cubes until smooth.

Usage:

Drink this curcumin smoothie in the morning or as a snack to benefit from its anti-inflammatory properties and support cellular health.

Benefits:

Curcumin helps reduce inflammation and supports cellular health, potentially aiding in the prevention of prostate cancer. Combined with other nutritious ingredients, this smoothie promotes overall well-being.

321. Aloe Vera Detox Juice

Description:

Aloe Vera juice promotes digestion and helps detoxify the body, which is crucial for maintaining hormonal balance.

Ingredients:

- 1/4 cup fresh aloe vera gel (from the inner leaf)
- 1 cup water or fresh juice (such as orange or apple juice)

□ 1 tablespoon honey (optional for sweetness)

Preparation Steps:

1. Scoop the fresh aloe vera gel from the inner leaf.

2. Blend the aloe vera gel with water or juice until smooth.

3. Add honey if desired for sweetness.

Usage:

Drink this aloe vera juice daily, preferably in the morning, to help detoxify the body and support digestive health.

Benefits:

Aloe Vera aids in digestion and detoxification, promoting hormonal balance and overall health. Regular consumption can help maintain a healthy digestive system and support the body's natural detox processes.

322. Vitamin B Complex Energy Smoothie

Description:

Vitamin B Complex is important for energy production and overall cellular metabolism, which are essential for maintaining men's health.

Ingredients:

□ 1 cup spinach (rich in B vitamins)

□ 1 banana

□ 1/2 cup Greek yogurt (rich in B12)

□ 1 cup fortified almond milk (contains B vitamins)

□ 1 tablespoon chia seeds

□ A handful of ice cubes

Preparation Steps:

Blend spinach, banana, Greek yogurt, fortified almond milk, chia seeds, and ice cubes until smooth.

Usage:

Drink this Vitamin B Complex energy smoothie in the morning to boost energy levels and support cellular metabolism.

Benefits:

This smoothie provides a rich source of B vitamins essential for energy production and cellular metabolism, promoting overall men's health and vitality.

323. Muira Puama Libido Boost Smoothie

Description:

Muira Puama, a Brazilian herb, is used to enhance sexual function and boost libido, making it a beneficial addition to a men's health smoothie.

Ingredients:

□ 1 teaspoon Muira Puama powder

□ 1 banana

□ 1 cup unsweetened almond milk

□ 1 tablespoon almond butter

□ 1 tablespoon honey (optional for sweetness)

□ A handful of ice cubes

Preparation Steps:

Blend Muira Puama powder, banana, almond milk, almond butter, honey, and ice cubes until smooth.

Usage:

Enjoy this Muira Puama libido boost smoothie in the morning or before an intimate evening to enhance sexual function and boost libido.

Benefits:

Muira Puama helps enhance sexual function and boost libido, while the other ingredients provide essential nutrients and energy, supporting overall men's health and vitality.

CHILDREN'S HEALTH REMEDIES

324. Elderberry Immune-Boosting Syrup

Description:

Elderberry syrup is known for its immune-boosting properties, helping to prevent and ease symptoms of colds and flu in children.

Ingredients:

- 1 cup fresh or dried elderberries
- 4 cups water
- 1 cup honey
- 1 teaspoon ground cinnamon (optional)
- 1 teaspoon ground ginger (optional)
- 1/2 teaspoon ground cloves (optional)

Preparation Steps:

1. Combine elderberries and water in a pot.
2. Bring to a boil, then reduce to a simmer for about 45 minutes, until the liquid reduces by half.
3. Remove from heat and let it cool.
4. Strain the mixture through a fine mesh strainer, pressing the berries to extract all the juice.
5. Stir in honey until well combined.
6. Pour the syrup into a glass jar and store in the refrigerator.

Usage:

Give children 1 teaspoon of elderberry syrup daily for immune support. Increase to 1 teaspoon every few hours if they show symptoms of a cold or flu.

Benefits:

Elderberry syrup boosts the immune system and helps reduce the duration and severity of colds and flu, supporting overall health and wellness in children.

325. Chamomile Calming Tea

Description:

Chamomile tea is a gentle herb that can calm anxiety, soothe stomach aches, and promote restful sleep for children.

Ingredients:

- 1 teaspoon dried chamomile flowers or 1 chamomile tea bag
- 1 cup boiling water
- Honey (optional, for sweetness)
- A slice of lemon (optional, for flavor)

Preparation Steps:

1. Steep chamomile flowers or tea bag in boiling water for 5-10 minutes.
2. Strain the tea and let it cool to a safe temperature for children.
3. Add honey and a slice of lemon if desired.

Usage:

Give children a cup of chamomile tea before bedtime or when they are feeling anxious or have an upset stomach.

Benefits:

Chamomile tea promotes relaxation, eases anxiety, soothes stomach aches, and helps children achieve restful sleep, supporting overall well-being.

326. Probiotic Yogurt

Parfait

Description:

Probiotics are essential for maintaining a healthy gut flora, aiding digestion, and boosting the immune system in children.

Ingredients:

- 1 cup plain Greek yogurt (rich in probiotics)
- 1/2 cup fresh berries (such as blueberries, strawberries, or raspberries)
- 1 tablespoon honey (optional for sweetness)
- 1/4 cup granola (for added texture and fiber)

Preparation Steps:

1. Layer the Greek yogurt in a bowl or glass.
2. Add fresh berries on top of the yogurt.
3. Drizzle with honey if desired.
4. Sprinkle granola over the berries.

Usage:

Serve this probiotic yogurt parfait as a breakfast or snack to support digestive health and boost the immune system.

Benefits:

Probiotics in Greek yogurt help maintain a healthy gut microbiome, essential for digestion and immune function. The added berries and granola provide fiber, vitamins, and antioxidants, enhancing overall health.

327. Vitamin D-Fortified Smoothie

Description:

Vitamin D is important for bone growth and immune function, especially in regions with limited sunlight exposure.

Ingredients:

- 1 cup fortified orange juice (rich in vitamin D)
- 1 banana
- 1/2 cup Greek yogurt (additional source of vitamin D and calcium)
- 1 tablespoon chia seeds
- A handful of ice cubes

Preparation Steps:

Blend fortified orange juice, banana, Greek yogurt, chia seeds, and ice cubes until smooth.

Usage:

Give children this vitamin D-fortified smoothie in the morning to ensure they get a good dose of this crucial nutrient for bone health and immune support.

Benefits:

Fortified orange juice and Greek yogurt provide vitamin D, essential for strong bones and a healthy immune system. This smoothie is a delicious way to help children meet their daily vitamin D needs.

328. Fish Oil Omega-3 Gummies

Description:

Fish oil is rich in omega-3 fatty acids, which are crucial for brain development and can improve attention in children.

Ingredients:

- 1/2 cup fish oil (liquid form, flavored for better taste)
- 1/2 cup fresh orange juice
- 1 tablespoon honey (optional for sweetness)
- 3 tablespoons gelatin powder

Preparation Steps:

1. Heat the orange juice in a small saucepan over low heat.

2. Stir in the honey and gelatin powder until fully dissolved.

3. Remove from heat and let it cool slightly.

4. Stir in the fish oil until well combined.

5. Pour the mixture into silicone molds and refrigerate until set.

Usage:

Give children 1-2 fish oil gummies daily to support brain development and improve attention.

Benefits:

Omega-3 fatty acids in fish oil are essential for cognitive development and can help improve focus and attention in children. These homemade gummies provide a tasty and convenient way to ensure kids get their daily dose of omega-3s.

329. Honey and Lemon Sore Throat Syrup

Description:

Honey and lemon are natural remedies for soothing sore throats and coughs. Note: Honey is only suitable for children over one year old.

Ingredients:

- 1/4 cup honey
- 1/4 cup fresh lemon juice (about 2 lemons)
- 1 cup warm water

Preparation Steps:

1. Mix honey and lemon juice in a cup of warm water until well combined.

Usage:

Give children 1-2 teaspoons of this honey and lemon syrup as needed to soothe sore throats and relieve coughs.

Benefits:

Honey provides a soothing coating for the throat, while lemon juice offers vitamin C and antioxidants to support the immune system. This combination helps alleviate throat irritation and coughs.

330. Aloe Vera Skin Soother Gel

Description:

Aloe Vera can be applied topically to soothe skin irritations such as sunburns or minor scrapes.

Ingredients:

- 1/4 cup fresh aloe vera gel (from the inner leaf)
- A few drops of lavender essential oil (optional for added soothing effects)

Preparation Steps:

1. Scoop the fresh aloe vera gel from the inner leaf.

2. Mix with a few drops of lavender essential oil if desired.

Usage:

Apply the aloe vera gel directly to the affected skin area to soothe irritation and promote healing.

Benefits:

Aloe Vera provides immediate cooling relief and helps speed up the healing process for sunburns, minor scrapes, and other skin irritations. Lavender oil adds extra soothing properties and a pleasant scent.

331. Flaxseed Oil Brain Boost Smoothie

Description:

Flaxseed oil is a plant-based source of omega-3s, beneficial for brain health and overall growth in children.

Ingredients:

- 1 tablespoon flaxseed oil
- 1 banana
- 1 cup unsweetened almond milk
- 1/2 cup frozen berries (such as blueberries or strawberries)
- 1 tablespoon honey (optional for sweetness)
- A handful of ice cubes

Preparation Steps:

1. Blend flaxseed oil, banana, almond milk, frozen berries, honey, and ice cubes until smooth.

Usage:

Serve this flaxseed oil brain boost smoothie as a nutritious breakfast or snack to support brain health and overall development.

Benefits:

Flaxseed oil provides omega-3 fatty acids, essential for cognitive development and overall growth. This smoothie combines nutrient-dense ingredients to promote brain health and vitality in children.

332. Echinacea Immune-Boosting Tea

Description:

Echinacea can help boost the immune system when taken at the onset of a cold, making it a valuable remedy for children's health.

Ingredients:

- 1 teaspoon dried echinacea leaves or 1 echinacea tea bag
- 1 cup boiling water
- Honey (optional for sweetness)
- Lemon wedge (optional for flavor)

Preparation Steps:

1. Steep dried echinacea leaves or tea bag in boiling water for 5-10 minutes.

2. Strain the tea and let it cool to a safe temperature for children.

3. Add honey and a lemon wedge if desired.

Usage:

Give children a cup of echinacea tea at the first sign of a cold to help boost their immune system.

Benefits:

Echinacea tea supports immune function, potentially reducing the severity and duration of colds. Honey and lemon add flavor and additional immune-boosting properties.

333. Peppermint Digestive Relief Tea

Description:

Peppermint tea relieves digestive problems such as gas and indigestion and can be a mild, soothing option for children.

Ingredients:

- 1 teaspoon dried peppermint leaves or 1 peppermint tea bag
- 1 cup boiling water
- Honey (optional for sweetness)

Preparation Steps:

1. Steep dried peppermint leaves or tea bag in boiling water for 5-10 minutes.

2. Strain the tea and let it cool to a safe temperature for children.

3. Add honey if desired.

Usage:

Give children a cup of peppermint tea after meals or when they experience digestive discomfort.

Benefits:

Peppermint tea helps soothe the digestive tract, relieving symptoms of gas and indigestion. Its mild flavor makes it an appealing choice for children.

334. Calendula Healing Cream

Description:

Calendula cream is ideal for treating diaper rashes, minor cuts, and scrapes due to its soothing and healing properties.

Ingredients:

- 1/4 cup dried calendula flowers
- 1/2 cup coconut oil
- 1/4 cup shea butter
- 1/4 cup beeswax

Preparation Steps:

1. Melt the coconut oil, shea butter, and beeswax in a double boiler.
2. Add the dried calendula flowers and let them infuse in the melted mixture for 1 hour on low heat.
3. Strain the mixture through a cheesecloth to remove the flowers.
4. Pour the mixture into a jar and let it cool and solidify.

Usage:

Apply calendula cream to diaper rashes, minor cuts, and scrapes as needed to soothe and heal the skin.

Benefits:

Calendula cream has anti-inflammatory and antiseptic properties, making it effective for healing skin irritations and promoting faster recovery.

335. Zinc Lozenges for Cold Relief

Description:

Zinc lozenges can reduce the duration of colds when taken at the first sign of symptoms, providing relief and supporting immune health.

Usage:

Give children zinc lozenges as directed on the packaging, typically one lozenge every 2-3 hours at the first sign of a cold.

Benefits:

Zinc helps support the immune system and can shorten the duration of colds. Lozenges provide an easy and effective way to administer zinc for cold relief.

336. Arnica Pain Relief Gel

Description:

Arnica gel is used for pain relief from bruises, sprains, and sore muscles, suitable for children after minor injuries.

Usage:

Apply a small amount of arnica gel to the affected area and gently massage it in. Use 2-3 times a day as needed.

Benefits:

Arnica gel helps reduce inflammation and pain, speeding up the healing process for bruises, sprains, and sore muscles. It's a gentle and effective remedy for minor injuries.

337. Lavender Sleep Aid Aromatherapy

Description:

Lavender essential oil is used in aromatherapy to help reduce anxiety and promote sleep at bedtime.

Ingredients:

- A few drops of lavender essential oil
- A diffuser or a bowl of hot water

Preparation Steps:

1. Add a few drops of lavender essential oil to a diffuser or a bowl of hot water.

Usage:

Place the diffuser or bowl in the child's bedroom about 30 minutes before bedtime to fill the room with a calming scent.

Benefits:

Lavender oil helps reduce anxiety and promotes relaxation, making it easier for children to fall asleep and enjoy a restful night.

338. Mullein Ear Oil for Ear Pain

Description:

Mullein ear oil is a traditional remedy used to relieve ear pain associated with ear infections.

Ingredients:

- 1/4 cup dried mullein flowers
- 1/4 cup olive oil
- 1 clove garlic (optional, for added antibacterial properties)

Preparation Steps:

1. Warm the olive oil in a double boiler.
2. Add the dried mullein flowers (and garlic if using) and let them infuse on low heat for 1 hour.
3. Strain the oil through a cheesecloth into a dropper bottle.

Usage:

Warm the oil to body temperature and apply 2-3 drops into the affected ear, allowing the child to lie still for a few minutes to let the oil penetrate.

Benefits:

Mullein ear oil helps reduce inflammation and pain in the ear, providing relief from ear infections and promoting healing.

339. Banana Recovery Smoothie

Description:

Bananas are easily digestible and rich in potassium, making them great for children, especially during recovery from stomach flu.

Ingredients:

- 1 banana
- 1 cup unsweetened almond milk
- 1 tablespoon honey (optional, for sweetness)
- A handful of ice cubes

Preparation Steps:

1. Blend the banana, almond milk, honey, and ice cubes until smooth.

Usage:

Serve this banana smoothie to children recovering from stomach flu to help replenish nutrients and provide gentle nourishment.

Benefits:

Bananas are rich in potassium and easy to digest, making them ideal for recovery from stomach ailments. This smoothie helps restore electrolytes and energy.

340. Oatmeal Soothing Bath

Description:

Oatmeal baths soothe itchy skin and can be very comforting for conditions like chickenpox or eczema.

Ingredients:

- 1 cup colloidal oatmeal or finely ground oatmeal
- Warm bathwater

Preparation Steps:

1. Add the colloidal oatmeal to warm bathwater and stir until it is evenly dispersed.

Usage:

Let the child soak in the oatmeal bath for 15-20 minutes to relieve itching and soothe irritated skin.

Benefits:

Oatmeal baths provide relief from itching and irritation caused by conditions like chickenpox or eczema, promoting skin healing and comfort.

341. Ginger Lollipops for Nausea Relief

Description:

Ginger can help reduce nausea, and ginger lollipops are a child-friendly way to alleviate motion sickness.

Ingredients:

- 1/2 cup fresh ginger root, peeled and sliced
- 2 cups water
- 1 cup sugar
- 1/4 cup light corn syrup
- Lollipop sticks
- Candy thermometer

Preparation Steps:

1. Boil the ginger slices in water for about 30 minutes, then strain to make ginger tea.
2. Combine the ginger tea, sugar, and corn syrup in a pot. Heat over medium-high until the mixture reaches 300°F on a candy thermometer.
3. Remove from heat and pour into lollipop molds, placing sticks in each mold.
4. Let the lollipops cool and harden.

Usage:

Give children a ginger lollipop as needed to help reduce nausea and motion sickness.

Benefits:

Ginger helps soothe nausea and is an effective natural remedy for motion sickness, making these lollipops a tasty and practical solution for kids.

342. Rice Water for Diarrhea Treatment

Description:

Rice water is effective in treating diarrhea in children by replenishing fluids and nutrients lost during illness.

Ingredients:

- 1 cup white rice
- 4 cups water

Preparation Steps:

Boil the rice in water for about 20 minutes, then strain the liquid into a clean container.

Usage:

Let the rice water cool, then give children small amounts to drink throughout the day to help treat diarrhea.

Benefits:

Rice water helps rehydrate and replenish lost nutrients, providing a gentle and effective way to treat diarrhea in children.

343. Coconut Water for Hydration

Description:

Coconut water is a natural hydration solution rich in electrolytes, ideal for rehydrating after physical activity or mild illness.

Ingredients:

- 1 cup fresh coconut water
- 1 tablespoon honey (optional, for sweetness)
- Preparation Steps:
- Mix coconut water and honey if desired.

Usage:

Serve chilled coconut water to children after physical activity or during mild illness to help rehydrate.

Benefits:

Coconut water is rich in electrolytes, making it an excellent natural hydration solution that helps replenish fluids and maintain electrolyte balance.

344. Slippery Elm Digestive Relief

Description:

Slippery Elm can be used for digestive issues; it coats the digestive tract, soothing an upset stomach.

Ingredients:

- 1 teaspoon slippery elm powder
- 1 cup warm water
- Honey (optional, for sweetness)

Preparation Steps:

1. Mix slippery elm powder with warm water until it forms a smooth mixture.
2. Add honey if desired.

Usage:

Give children this slippery elm mixture to drink when they have an upset stomach.

Benefits:

Slippery Elm coats and soothes the digestive tract, providing relief from digestive discomfort and upset stomachs.

345. Cranberry Juice for UTI Prevention

Description:

Cranberry juice helps prevent urinary tract infections (UTIs), which are relatively common in young children.

Ingredients:

- 1 cup pure cranberry juice (unsweetened)
- 1 cup water
- Honey (optional, for sweetness)

Preparation Steps:

1. Dilute the cranberry juice with water.
2. Add honey if desired for sweetness.

Usage:

Give children a cup of diluted cranberry juice daily to help prevent UTIs.

Benefits:

Cranberry juice helps prevent bacteria from adhering to the urinary tract walls, reducing the risk of UTIs in children. Regular consumption supports urinary tract health.

346. Almond Milk Calcium Boost Smoothie

Description:

Almond milk is a dairy-free alternative rich in calcium and vitamin E, suitable for children with lactose intolerance.

Ingredients:

- 1 cup unsweetened almond milk
- 1 banana
- 1/2 cup spinach (for added nutrients)
- 1 tablespoon almond butter
- 1 tablespoon honey (optional, for sweetness)
- A handful of ice cubes

Preparation Steps:

1. Blend almond milk, banana, spinach, almond butter, honey, and ice cubes until smooth.

Usage:

Serve this almond milk smoothie as a nutritious breakfast or snack to provide calcium and vitamin E.

Benefits:

Almond milk is a great source of calcium and vitamin E, supporting bone health and overall well-being in children with lactose intolerance.

347. Baking Soda Itch Relief Paste

Description:

A paste made from baking soda and water can relieve itching from insect bites or poison ivy.

Ingredients:

- 2 tablespoons baking soda
- Enough water to make a thick paste

Preparation Steps:

1. Mix baking soda with water to form a thick paste.

Usage:

Apply the baking soda paste to insect bites or areas affected by poison ivy. Let it sit for a few minutes, then rinse off with cool water. Repeat as needed.

Benefits:

Baking soda helps neutralize the itch and soothe irritated skin, providing relief from insect bites and poison ivy.

348. Tart Cherry Sleep Aid Juice

Description:

Tart cherry juice contains natural melatonin, which can help regulate sleep cycles in children having trouble sleeping.

Ingredients:

- 1 cup tart cherry juice (unsweetened)
- 1 cup water
- Honey (optional, for sweetness)

Preparation Steps:

1. Dilute the tart cherry juice with water.
2. Add honey if desired for sweetness.

Usage:

Give children a cup of diluted tart cherry juice about 30 minutes before bedtime to help regulate sleep.

Benefits:

Tart cherry juice provides natural melatonin, helping to regulate sleep cycles and improve sleep quality in children. Regular consumption can support better sleep habits and overall health.

ELDERLY HEALTH REMEDIES

349. Ginkgo Biloba Cognitive Boost Tea

Description:

Ginkgo Biloba enhances cognitive function and circulation, commonly used to combat memory decline associated with aging.

Ingredients:

- 1 teaspoon dried Ginkgo Biloba leaves or 1 Ginkgo Biloba tea bag
- 1 cup boiling water
- Honey (optional, for sweetness)
- Lemon wedge (optional, for flavor)

Preparation Steps:

1. Steep the dried Ginkgo Biloba leaves or tea bag in boiling water for 5-10 minutes.
2. Strain the tea and let it cool to a safe drinking temperature.
3. Add honey and a lemon wedge if desired.

Usage:

Give elderly individuals a cup of Ginkgo Biloba tea daily to help enhance cognitive function and circulation.

Benefits:

Ginkgo Biloba supports improved memory and cognitive function, and enhances blood circulation, making it a beneficial remedy for combating age-related memory decline.

350. Omega-3 Fatty Acids Heart Health Smoothie

Description:

Omega-3 fatty acids are essential for maintaining cardiovascular health and reducing inflammation, crucial for elderly individuals.

Ingredients:

- 1 cup unsweetened almond milk
- 1 tablespoon flaxseed oil (rich in omega-3s)
- 1 banana
- 1/2 cup blueberries (additional antioxidants)
- 1 tablespoon chia seeds
- A handful of ice cubes

Preparation Steps:

Blend almond milk, flaxseed oil, banana, blueberries, chia seeds, and ice cubes until smooth.

Usage:

Serve this omega-3 rich smoothie as a nutritious breakfast or snack to support heart health and reduce inflammation.

Benefits:

Omega-3 fatty acids help maintain cardiovascular health and reduce inflammation, promoting overall well-being in elderly individuals.

351. Turmeric Anti-Inflammatory Golden Milk

Description:

Turmeric has potent anti-inflammatory properties that help reduce symptoms of arthritis and other inflammatory conditions prevalent in elderly populations.

Ingredients:

- 1 teaspoon turmeric powder
- 1 cup unsweetened almond milk
- 1/2 teaspoon cinnamon
- 1 tablespoon honey (optional, for sweetness)
- A pinch of black pepper (enhances curcumin absorption)

Preparation Steps:

1. Heat the almond milk in a saucepan over medium heat.
2. Add turmeric powder, cinnamon, honey, and

black pepper, and stir well.

3. Simmer for a few minutes, then let it cool to a safe drinking temperature.

Usage:

Give elderly individuals a cup of turmeric golden milk daily to help reduce inflammation and joint pain.

Benefits:

Turmeric helps reduce inflammation and pain associated with arthritis and other inflammatory conditions, supporting joint and muscle health.

352. Ginger Tea for Digestive Health

Description:

Ginger tea aids digestion and relieves nausea, while also having anti-inflammatory effects that can help with joint and muscle pain.

Ingredients:

- 1-2 inches fresh ginger root, peeled and sliced
- 1 cup boiling water
- Honey (optional, for sweetness)
- Lemon wedge (optional, for flavor)

Preparation Steps:

1. Steep the sliced ginger root in boiling water for 10-15 minutes.

2. Strain the tea and let it cool to a safe drinking temperature.

3. Add honey and a lemon wedge if desired.

Usage:

Serve ginger tea to elderly individuals after meals or when experiencing digestive discomfort.

Benefits:

Ginger tea promotes digestive health, relieves nausea, and has anti-inflammatory properties

that help reduce joint and muscle pain.

353. Hawthorn Berry Heart Health Tea

Description:

Hawthorn Berry supports heart health by improving blood flow and strengthening heart muscles, ideal for managing heart conditions in older adults.

Ingredients:

- 1 teaspoon dried hawthorn berries
- 1 cup boiling water
- Honey (optional, for sweetness)
- Lemon wedge (optional, for flavor)

Preparation Steps:

1. Steep the dried hawthorn berries in boiling water for 10-15 minutes.

2. Strain the tea and let it cool to a safe drinking temperature.

3. Add honey and a lemon wedge if desired.

Usage:

Give elderly individuals a cup of hawthorn berry tea daily to support heart health and improve blood flow.

Benefits:

Hawthorn Berry tea helps improve cardiovascular function, supports healthy blood flow, and strengthens the heart muscles, making it beneficial for managing heart conditions in older adults.

354. Probiotic Gut Health Smoothie

Description:

Probiotics are essential for gut health, which is vital for immune function and nutrient absorption, especially critical in the elderly.

Ingredients:

- 1 cup plain Greek yogurt (rich in probiotics)
- 1/2 cup fresh berries (such as blueberries or strawberries)
- 1 banana
- 1 tablespoon honey (optional for sweetness)
- 1/4 cup granola (for added fiber and texture)

Preparation Steps:

1. Blend Greek yogurt, berries, banana, and honey until smooth.
2. Top with granola for added crunch and fiber.

Usage:

Serve this probiotic smoothie as a nutritious breakfast or snack to support gut health and immune function.

Benefits:

Probiotics help maintain a healthy gut microbiome, essential for digestion, immune function, and overall health in elderly individuals.

355. Vitamin D3 Sunshine Smoothie

Description:

Vitamin D3 enhances bone density and immune function, addressing common deficiencies in elderly individuals due to less exposure to sunlight.

Ingredients:

- 1 cup fortified orange juice (rich in vitamin D)
- 1 banana
- 1/2 cup Greek yogurt (additional source of vitamin D and calcium)
- 1 tablespoon chia seeds (for added nutrients)
- A handful of ice cubes

Preparation Steps:

1. Blend fortified orange juice, banana, Greek yogurt, chia seeds, and ice cubes until smooth.

Usage:

Serve this vitamin D3 smoothie in the morning to boost vitamin D levels and support bone health and immune function.

Benefits:

Vitamin D3 is crucial for bone health and immune function, helping to address deficiencies and promote overall well-being in elderly individuals.

356. Calcium Bone Health 357. Smoothie

Description:

Calcium is crucial for maintaining bone health to prevent osteoporosis and fractures.

Ingredients:

- 1 cup unsweetened almond milk (fortified with calcium)
- 1/2 cup Greek yogurt (rich in calcium)
- 1 banana
- 1 tablespoon almond butter
- A handful of ice cubes

Preparation Steps:

Blend almond milk, Greek yogurt, banana, almond butter, and ice cubes until smooth.

Usage:

Serve this calcium-rich smoothie as a daily drink to support bone health and prevent osteoporosis.

Benefits:

Calcium is essential for maintaining strong bones, preventing osteoporosis, and reducing the risk of fractures in elderly individuals.

358. Adaptogenic Herbs Resilience Tea

Description:

Adaptogenic herbs like ashwagandha and rhodiola help the body manage stress and reduce fatigue, enhancing overall resilience in the elderly.

Ingredients:

- 1 teaspoon ashwagandha powder
- 1 teaspoon rhodiola powder
- 1 cup boiling water
- Honey (optional, for sweetness)

Preparation Steps:

1. Steep ashwagandha and rhodiola powders in boiling water for 5-10 minutes.
2. Strain the tea and let it cool to a safe drinking temperature.
3. Add honey if desired.

Usage:

Serve this adaptogenic tea once daily to help manage stress and reduce fatigue.

Benefits:

Adaptogenic herbs help the body adapt to stress, reduce fatigue, and enhance overall resilience, promoting better mental and physical health in elderly individuals.

359. Magnesium Relaxation Drink

Description:

Magnesium promotes muscle and nerve function, helps regulate heart rhythms, and improves sleep, all important for elderly health.

Ingredients:

- 1 cup warm water
- 1 tablespoon magnesium citrate powder
- Honey and lemon (optional, for flavor)

Preparation Steps:

1. Mix magnesium citrate powder with warm water until dissolved.
2. Add honey and lemon if desired for taste.

Usage:

Drink this magnesium relaxation drink in the evening to promote muscle and nerve function, regulate heart rhythms, and improve sleep.

Benefits:

Magnesium supports muscle and nerve function, heart health, and sleep quality, making it a vital nutrient for elderly health and well-being.

360. Green Tea Antioxidant Smoothie

Description:

Green tea is rich in antioxidants that help protect against cellular damage and reduce the risk of chronic diseases like heart disease and cancer.

Ingredients:

- 1 cup brewed green tea, cooled
- 1 banana
- 1/2 cup spinach
- 1/2 cup Greek yogurt
- 1 tablespoon honey (optional for sweetness)
- A handful of ice cubes

Preparation Steps:

1. Brew green tea and let it cool.
2. Blend the cooled green tea, banana, spinach, Greek yogurt, honey, and ice cubes until smooth.

Usage:

Enjoy this green tea antioxidant smoothie in the morning or as an afternoon pick-me-up to boost your antioxidant intake and support overall health.

Benefits:

Green tea provides powerful antioxidants that protect against cellular damage, reducing the risk of chronic diseases and promoting overall health in elderly individuals.

361. Coenzyme Q10 Energy Boost Smoothie

Description:

Coenzyme Q10 supports energy production in cells and has antioxidant properties, which are important for aging bodies.

Ingredients:

- 1 teaspoon Coenzyme Q10 powder or liquid
- 1 cup unsweetened almond milk
- 1 banana
- 1/2 cup Greek yogurt
- 1 tablespoon honey (optional for sweetness)
- A handful of ice cubes

Preparation Steps:

Blend Coenzyme Q10, almond milk, banana, Greek yogurt, honey, and ice cubes until smooth.

Usage:

Enjoy this Coenzyme Q10 energy boost smoothie in the morning to support cellular energy production and overall vitality.

Benefits:

Coenzyme Q10 enhances energy production at the cellular level and provides antioxidant protection, supporting overall health and energy levels in elderly individuals.

362. Saw Palmetto Prostate Health Tea

Description:

Saw Palmetto is beneficial for prostate health and in managing symptoms of benign prostatic hyperplasia (BPH) in elderly men.

Ingredients:

- 1 teaspoon dried Saw Palmetto berries or 1 Saw Palmetto tea bag
- 1 cup boiling water
- Honey (optional, for sweetness)
- Lemon wedge (optional, for flavor)

Preparation Steps:

1. Steep the dried Saw Palmetto berries or tea bag in boiling water for 10-15 minutes.
2. Strain the tea and let it cool to a safe drinking temperature.
3. Add honey and a lemon wedge if desired.

Usage:

Give elderly men a cup of Saw Palmetto tea daily to support prostate health and manage BPH symptoms.

Benefits:

Saw Palmetto helps reduce symptoms of BPH, such as frequent urination, and supports overall prostate health, improving quality of life for elderly men.

363. Bilberry Eye Health Smoothie

Description:

Bilberry extract enhances eye health and circulation, helping to prevent age-related macular degeneration.

Ingredients:

- 1 teaspoon bilberry extract
- 1 cup unsweetened almond milk
- 1/2 cup blueberries (additional antioxidants)
- 1 banana
- 1 tablespoon honey (optional for sweetness)
- A handful of ice cubes

Preparation Steps:

1. Blend bilberry extract, almond milk, blueberries, banana, honey, and ice cubes until smooth.

Usage:

Enjoy this bilberry eye health smoothie as a nutritious breakfast or snack to support eye health and circulation.

Benefits:

Bilberry extract and blueberries are rich in antioxidants that support eye health and improve circulation, helping to prevent age-related macular degeneration and maintain vision.

364. Lavender Aromatherapy for Relaxation

Description:

Lavender oil is used in aromatherapy to help reduce anxiety, promote relaxation, and aid in sleep, which can be problematic for the elderly.

Ingredients:

- A few drops of lavender essential oil
- A diffuser or a bowl of hot water

Preparation Steps:

Add a few drops of lavender essential oil to a diffuser or a bowl of hot water.

Usage:

Place the diffuser or bowl in the bedroom about 30 minutes before bedtime to fill the room with a calming scent. Use as needed to help reduce anxiety and promote relaxation.

Benefits:

Lavender oil helps reduce anxiety, promotes relaxation, and aids in sleep, making it beneficial for elderly individuals who may struggle with sleep issues.

365. Rosemary Brain Boost Tea

Description:

Rosemary boosts brain function and circulation, and can enhance memory and focus, making it a beneficial herb for elderly individuals.

Ingredients:

- 1 teaspoon dried rosemary leaves or 1 rosemary tea bag
- 1 cup boiling water
- Honey (optional, for sweetness)
- Lemon wedge (optional, for flavor)

Preparation Steps:

1. Steep the dried rosemary leaves or tea bag in boiling water for 5-10 minutes.
2. Strain the tea and let it cool to a safe drinking temperature.
3. Add honey and a lemon wedge if desired.

Usage:

Drink a cup of rosemary tea daily to support brain function, enhance memory, and improve circulation.

Benefits:

Rosemary tea helps boost cognitive function, memory, and focus, supporting overall brain health and circulation in elderly individuals.

366. Nettle Tea for Joint Health

Description:

Nettle tea is rich in nutrients important for joint health and reducing inflammation, and also supports kidney function.

Ingredients:

- 1 teaspoon dried nettle leaves or 1 nettle tea bag
- 1 cup boiling water
- Honey (optional, for sweetness)
- Lemon wedge (optional, for flavor)

Preparation Steps:

1. Steep the dried nettle leaves or tea bag in boiling water for 10-15 minutes.
2. Strain the tea and let it cool to a safe drinking temperature.
3. Add honey and a lemon wedge if desired.

Usage:

Drink a cup of nettle tea daily to support joint health, reduce inflammation, and promote kidney function.

Benefits:

Nettle tea provides essential nutrients for joint health, reduces inflammation, and supports kidney function, enhancing overall well-being in elderly individuals.

367. Flaxseed Heart Health Smoothie

Description:

Flaxseeds are high in omega-3 fatty acids and fiber, beneficial for heart health and maintaining regular bowel movements.

Ingredients:

- 1 tablespoon ground flaxseeds
- 1 banana
- 1 cup unsweetened almond milk
- 1/2 cup frozen berries (such as blueberries or strawberries)
- 1 tablespoon honey (optional, for sweetness)
- A handful of ice cubes

Preparation Steps:

1. Blend ground flaxseeds, banana, almond milk, frozen berries, honey, and ice cubes until smooth.

Usage:

Enjoy this flaxseed heart health smoothie in the morning or as a snack to support heart health and digestive regularity.

Benefits:

Flaxseeds provide omega-3 fatty acids and fiber, which support heart health and promote regular bowel movements, essential for maintaining overall health in elderly individuals.

368. Garlic Cardiovascular Health Tonic

Description:

Garlic helps lower blood pressure and cholesterol levels, supporting cardiovascular health in elderly individuals.

Ingredients:

- 2-3 cloves of fresh garlic, minced
- 1 cup warm water
- Honey (optional, for sweetness)
- Lemon juice (optional, for flavor)

Preparation Steps:

1. Mix minced garlic with warm water.

2. Add honey and lemon juice if desired for better taste.

Usage:

Drink this garlic tonic daily to support cardiovascular health and lower blood pressure and cholesterol levels.

Benefits:

Garlic has natural properties that help lower blood pressure and cholesterol, promoting cardiovascular health and reducing the risk of heart disease.

369. Peppermint Digestive Relief Tea

Description:

Peppermint alleviates digestive problems such as gas, bloating, and indigestion, common in elderly individuals.

Ingredients:

- 1 teaspoon dried peppermint leaves or 1 peppermint tea bag
- 1 cup boiling water
- Honey (optional, for sweetness)

Preparation Steps:

1. Steep the dried peppermint leaves or tea bag in boiling water for 5-10 minutes.

2. Strain the tea and let it cool to a safe drinking temperature.

3. Add honey if desired.

Usage:

Drink a cup of peppermint tea after meals or when experiencing digestive discomfort to alleviate symptoms.

Benefits:

Peppermint tea helps soothe the digestive tract, relieving gas, bloating, and indigestion, promoting better digestive health in elderly individuals.

370. Chamomile Calming Tea

Description:

Chamomile has calming effects that help manage sleep disorders and provide a soothing effect on the digestive system, supporting overall longevity.

Ingredients:

- 1 teaspoon dried chamomile flowers or 1 chamomile tea bag
- 1 cup boiling water
- Honey (optional, for sweetness)
- Lemon wedge (optional, for flavor)

Preparation Steps:

1. Steep the dried chamomile flowers or tea bag in boiling water for 5-10 minutes.

2. Strain the tea and let it cool to a safe drinking temperature.

3. Add honey and a lemon wedge if desired.

Usage:

Drink a cup of chamomile tea before bedtime to promote restful sleep and soothe the digestive system.

Benefits:

Chamomile tea promotes relaxation, aids in sleep, and soothes the digestive tract, contributing to better sleep quality and digestive health for longevity.

371. Aloe Vera Digestive Health Juice

Description:

Aloe Vera juice promotes healthy digestion and can relieve constipation, a common issue in the elderly, aiding in longevity.

Ingredients:

- 1/4 cup fresh aloe vera gel (from the inner leaf)
- 1 cup water or fresh juice (such as orange or apple juice)
- 1 tablespoon honey (optional for sweetness)

Preparation Steps:

1. Scoop the fresh aloe vera gel from the inner leaf.
2. Blend the aloe vera gel with water or juice until smooth.
3. Add honey if desired for sweetness.

Usage:

Drink this aloe vera juice daily, preferably in the morning, to support healthy digestion and relieve constipation.

Benefits:

Aloe Vera aids in digestion and helps alleviate constipation, promoting a healthy digestive system which is crucial for longevity.

372. Slippery Elm Digestive Soother

Description:

Slippery Elm is useful for treating acid reflux and soothing the digestive tract, providing relief from gastrointestinal discomfort, contributing to longevity.

Ingredients:

- 1 teaspoon slippery elm powder
- 1 cup warm water
- Honey (optional, for sweetness)

Preparation Steps:

1. Mix slippery elm powder with warm water until it forms a smooth mixture.
2. Add honey if desired.

Usage:

Drink this slippery elm mixture when experiencing acid reflux or gastrointestinal discomfort to soothe the digestive tract.

Benefits:

Slippery Elm helps coat and soothe the digestive tract, relieving acid reflux and gastrointestinal discomfort, supporting digestive health for longevity.

373. Cranberry UTI Prevention Juice

Description:

Cranberry juice prevents urinary tract infections, which are more prevalent in elderly populations, especially in women, supporting longevity.

Ingredients:

- 1 cup pure cranberry juice (unsweetened)
- 1 cup water
- Honey (optional, for sweetness)

Preparation Steps:

1. Dilute the cranberry juice with water.
2. Add honey if desired for sweetness.

Usage:

Drink a cup of diluted cranberry juice daily to help prevent urinary tract infections.

Benefits:

Cranberry juice helps prevent bacteria from adhering to the urinary tract walls, reducing the risk of UTIs and promoting urinary tract health, contributing to longevity.

374. Licorice Root Gastrointestinal Relief Tea

Description:

Licorice root helps in managing gastrointestinal issues and can soothe stomach ulcers and indigestion, supporting overall longevity.

Ingredients:

- 1 teaspoon dried licorice root
- 1 cup boiling water
- Honey (optional, for sweetness)

Preparation Steps:

1. Steep the dried licorice root in boiling water for 10-15 minutes.
2. Strain the tea and let it cool to a safe drinking temperature.
3. Add honey if desired.

Usage:

Drink a cup of licorice root tea when experiencing gastrointestinal discomfort or indigestion.

Benefits:

Licorice root helps soothe stomach ulcers and indigestion, providing relief from gastrointestinal issues and promoting digestive health, which is essential for longevity.

MENTAL CLARITY AND FOCUS REMEDIES

375. Rhodiola Rosea Concentration Tea

Description:

Rhodiola Rosea helps improve concentration and reduce mental fatigue, particularly useful during stressful periods.

Ingredients:

- 1 teaspoon dried Rhodiola Rosea root or 1 Rhodiola Rosea tea bag
- 1 cup boiling water
- Honey (optional, for sweetness)
- Lemon wedge (optional, for flavor)

Preparation Steps:

1. Steep the dried Rhodiola Rosea root or tea bag in boiling water for 10-15 minutes.
2. Strain the tea and let it cool to a safe drinking temperature.
3. Add honey and a lemon wedge if desired.

Usage:

Drink a cup of Rhodiola Rosea tea during periods of stress to enhance concentration and reduce mental fatigue.

Benefits:

Rhodiola Rosea tea supports improved concentration and reduces mental fatigue, promoting better mental clarity and focus during stressful times.

376. Phosphatidylserine Brain Function Smoothie

Description:

Phosphatidylserine covers and protects the cells in your brain and carries messages between them, helping to enhance memory and cognitive capacity.

Ingredients:

- 1 teaspoon phosphatidylserine powder
- 1 cup unsweetened almond milk
- 1 banana

- 1/2 cup Greek yogurt
- 1 tablespoon honey (optional, for sweetness)
- A handful of ice cubes

Preparation Steps:

Blend phosphatidylserine powder, almond milk, banana, Greek yogurt, honey, and ice cubes until smooth.

Usage:

Enjoy this phosphatidylserine smoothie in the morning to support brain function and enhance memory.

Benefits:

Phosphatidylserine helps protect brain cells and enhance cognitive capacity, contributing to improved memory and mental performance.

377. Acetyl-L-Carnitine Energy Boost Drink

Description:

Acetyl-L-Carnitine is known for its role in producing energy and its ability to increase alertness, focus, and mental clarity.

Ingredients:

- 1 teaspoon Acetyl-L-Carnitine powder
- 1 cup unsweetened almond milk
- 1 banana
- 1 tablespoon almond butter
- 1 tablespoon honey (optional, for sweetness)
- A handful of ice cubes

Preparation Steps:

1. Blend Acetyl-L-Carnitine powder, almond milk, banana, almond butter, honey, and ice cubes until smooth.

Usage:

Drink this Acetyl-L-Carnitine energy boost drink

in the morning to enhance alertness and mental clarity.

Benefits:

Acetyl-L-Carnitine helps produce energy and increases alertness and focus, promoting better mental clarity and cognitive function.

378. Caffeine with L-Theanine Focused Energy Tea

Description:

Caffeine combined with L-Theanine provides smooth and focused alertness without the jitteriness often associated with caffeine alone.

Ingredients:

- 1 cup brewed green tea (contains both caffeine and L-Theanine)
- 1 teaspoon matcha powder (optional, for an extra boost)
- Honey (optional, for sweetness)
- Lemon wedge (optional, for flavor)

Preparation Steps:

1. Brew green tea and let it cool to a safe drinking temperature.
2. Stir in matcha powder if desired.
3. Add honey and a lemon wedge if desired.

Usage:

Drink this green tea in the morning or afternoon for a smooth and focused energy boost.

Benefits:

The combination of caffeine and L-Theanine in green tea provides alertness and focus without jitteriness, supporting sustained mental performance and clarity.

379. Vitamin B Complex Brain Health Smoothie

Description:

Vitamin B Complex is essential for brain health and function, helping to reduce fatigue and improve mental performance.

Ingredients:

- 1 cup fortified almond milk (contains B vitamins)
- 1 banana
- 1/2 cup Greek yogurt (additional B vitamins)
- 1 tablespoon chia seeds
- A handful of ice cubes

Preparation Steps:

1. Blend fortified almond milk, banana, Greek yogurt, chia seeds, and ice cubes until smooth.

Usage:

Enjoy this Vitamin B Complex smoothie in the morning to support brain health and reduce fatigue.

Benefits:

B vitamins help reduce fatigue and improve mental performance, supporting overall brain health and function.

380. Huperzine A Memory Enhancer Tea

Description:

Huperzine A acts as a cholinesterase inhibitor, helping to increase levels of neurotransmitters in the brain, enhancing memory and protecting against cognitive decline.

Ingredients:

- 1 teaspoon Huperzine A powder

- 1 cup boiling water
- Honey (optional, for sweetness)
- Lemon wedge (optional, for flavor)

Preparation Steps:

1. Steep Huperzine A powder in boiling water for 10-15 minutes.
2. Strain the tea and let it cool to a safe drinking temperature.
3. Add honey and a lemon wedge if desired.

Usage:

Drink this Huperzine A tea daily to support memory and protect against cognitive decline.

Benefits:

Huperzine A helps enhance memory and cognitive function by increasing levels of neurotransmitters in the brain, promoting better mental clarity and focus.

381. Ashwagandha Stress-Relief Smoothie

Description:

Ashwagandha is an adaptogen that reduces stress and anxiety, thereby improving concentration and mental clarity.

Ingredients:

- 1 teaspoon ashwagandha powder
- 1 banana
- 1 cup unsweetened almond milk
- 1 tablespoon almond butter
- 1 tablespoon honey (optional, for sweetness)
- A handful of ice cubes

Preparation Steps:

Blend ashwagandha powder, banana, almond milk, almond butter, honey, and ice cubes until smooth.

Usage:

Drink this ashwagandha smoothie in the morning or as a midday snack to reduce stress and enhance concentration.

Benefits:

Ashwagandha helps lower stress and anxiety levels, promoting better concentration and mental clarity, supporting overall brain health and function.

382. Curcumin Brain Boost Smoothie

Description:

Curcumin, the active component in turmeric, has anti-inflammatory properties and boosts brain-derived neurotrophic factor (BDNF), supporting cognitive functions.

Ingredients:

- 1 teaspoon turmeric powder (curcumin)
- 1 banana
- 1 cup unsweetened almond milk
- 1/2 teaspoon black pepper (enhances curcumin absorption)
- 1 tablespoon honey (optional, for sweetness)
- A handful of ice cubes

Preparation Steps:

1. Blend turmeric powder, banana, almond milk, black pepper, honey, and ice cubes until smooth.

Usage:

Drink this curcumin smoothie in the morning to support brain health and cognitive function.

Benefits:

Curcumin has anti-inflammatory properties and boosts BDNF, enhancing cognitive functions and supporting overall brain health.

383. Matcha Green Tea Focus Drink

Description:

Matcha green tea contains high levels of L-theanine and a healthy dose of caffeine, which boost brain function and help maintain alertness.

Ingredients:

- 1 teaspoon matcha powder
- 1 cup hot water (not boiling)
- Honey (optional, for sweetness)
- Lemon wedge (optional, for flavor)

Preparation Steps:

1. Whisk matcha powder with hot water until frothy.
2. Add honey and a lemon wedge if desired.

Usage:

Drink this matcha green tea in the morning or early afternoon for a focused and alert state.

Benefits:

Matcha green tea combines caffeine and L-theanine to enhance brain function, maintaining alertness and promoting mental clarity.

384. Dark Chocolate Memory Booster Smoothie

Description:

Dark chocolate contains flavonoids that enhance memory and slow down cognitive decline, making it a delicious and beneficial addition to a smoothie.

Ingredients:

- 2 tablespoons cocoa powder (unsweetened)
- 1 banana
- 1 cup unsweetened almond milk

- 1 tablespoon honey (optional, for sweetness)
- A handful of ice cubes

Preparation Steps:

1. Blend cocoa powder, banana, almond milk, honey, and ice cubes until smooth.

Usage:

Enjoy this dark chocolate smoothie as a healthy treat to support memory and cognitive function.

Benefits:

Dark chocolate flavonoids enhance memory and slow cognitive decline, supporting overall brain health.

385. Sage Extract Memory Tea

Description:

Sage extract has been shown to improve memory recall and attention in several studies.

Ingredients:

- 1 teaspoon dried sage leaves or 1 sage tea bag
- 1 cup boiling water
- Honey (optional, for sweetness)
- Lemon wedge (optional, for flavor)

Preparation Steps:

1. Steep dried sage leaves or tea bag in boiling water for 10-15 minutes.
2. Strain the tea and let it cool to a safe drinking temperature.
3. Add honey and a lemon wedge if desired.

Usage:

Drink a cup of sage tea daily to improve memory recall and attention.

Benefits:

Sage extract enhances memory recall and attention, supporting better cognitive function and mental clarity.

386. Rosemary Essential Oil Inhalation

Description:

Rosemary essential oil inhalation can increase concentration and memory, historically associated with memory enhancement.

Ingredients:

- A few drops of rosemary essential oil
- A diffuser or a bowl of hot water

Preparation Steps:

1. Add a few drops of rosemary essential oil to a diffuser or a bowl of hot water.

Usage:

Inhale the rosemary-infused steam for a few minutes to boost concentration and memory.

Benefits:

Inhaling rosemary essential oil enhances concentration and memory, supporting cognitive function and mental clarity.

387. Gotu Kola Cognitive Function Tea

Description:

Gotu Kola is used in Ayurvedic and traditional Chinese medicine to improve cognitive function and reduce mental fatigue.

Ingredients:

- 1 teaspoon dried Gotu Kola leaves or 1 Gotu Kola tea bag
- 1 cup boiling water
- Honey (optional, for sweetness)

□ Lemon wedge (optional, for flavor)

Preparation Steps:

1. Steep dried Gotu Kola leaves or tea bag in boiling water for 10-15 minutes.

2. Strain the tea and let it cool to a safe drinking temperature.

3. Add honey and a lemon wedge if desired.

Usage:

Drink a cup of Gotu Kola tea daily to improve cognitive function and reduce mental fatigue.

Benefits:

Gotu Kola supports cognitive function, reduces mental fatigue, and promotes better mental clarity and focus.

388. Blueberry Brain Health Smoothie

Description:

Blueberries are high in antioxidants that may delay brain aging and improve overall cognitive function.

Ingredients:

□ 1 cup fresh or frozen blueberries

□ 1 banana

□ 1 cup unsweetened almond milk

□ 1/2 cup Greek yogurt

□ 1 tablespoon honey (optional, for sweetness)

□ A handful of ice cubes

Preparation Steps:

1. Blend blueberries, banana, almond milk, Greek yogurt, honey, and ice cubes until smooth.

Usage:

Enjoy this blueberry smoothie in the morning or as a snack to support brain health and cognitive function.

Benefits:

Blueberries provide powerful antioxidants that may help delay brain aging and improve cognitive function, promoting overall mental clarity and focus.

389. Pumpkin Seed Brain Boost Snack

Description:

Pumpkin seeds contain antioxidants and are rich in magnesium, iron, zinc, and copper, all essential for brain health.

Ingredients:

□ 1 cup raw pumpkin seeds

□ 1 tablespoon olive oil

□ Salt and pepper to taste

□ 1 teaspoon paprika (optional, for flavor)

Preparation Steps:

1. Toss pumpkin seeds with olive oil, salt, pepper, and paprika.

2. Spread seeds on a baking sheet and roast at 350°F (175°C) for 10-15 minutes, or until golden brown.

Usage:

Enjoy roasted pumpkin seeds as a snack to boost brain health.

Benefits:

Pumpkin seeds provide essential nutrients like magnesium, iron, zinc, and copper, supporting brain health and cognitive function.

390. MCT Oil Cognitive Performance Smoothie

Description:

MCT oil provides immediate fuel to the brain, enhancing cognitive performance and mental clarity.

Ingredients:
- 1 tablespoon MCT oil
- 1 cup unsweetened almond milk
- 1 banana
- 1 tablespoon cocoa powder (optional, for flavor)
- 1 tablespoon honey (optional, for sweetness)
- A handful of ice cubes

Preparation Steps:
1. Blend MCT oil, almond milk, banana, cocoa powder, honey, and ice cubes until smooth.

Usage:

Drink this MCT oil smoothie in the morning to enhance cognitive performance and mental clarity.

Benefits:

MCT oil provides quick energy to the brain, improving cognitive performance and supporting mental clarity throughout the day.

391. Kava Kava Calm Focus Tea

Description:

Kava Kava is known for its calming effects, which can help ease anxiety and improve focus during stressful situations.

Ingredients:
- 1 teaspoon kava kava powder
- 1 cup boiling water
- Honey (optional, for sweetness)
- Lemon wedge (optional, for flavor)

Preparation Steps:
1. Steep kava kava powder in boiling water for 10-15 minutes.
2. Strain the tea and let it cool to a safe drinking temperature.
3. Add honey and a lemon wedge if desired.

Usage:

Drink a cup of kava kava tea during stressful situations to ease anxiety and improve focus.

Benefits:

Kava kava tea provides calming effects, reducing anxiety and promoting better focus and mental clarity during stressful times.

392. Walnut Brain Health Snack

Description:

Walnuts are rich in alpha-linolenic acid, a plant-based omega-3 fatty acid, and other neuroprotective compounds that enhance brain health.

Ingredients:
- 1 cup raw walnuts
- 1 tablespoon olive oil
- Salt and pepper to taste
- 1 teaspoon rosemary (optional, for flavor)

Preparation Steps:
1. Toss walnuts with olive oil, salt, pepper, and rosemary.
2. Spread walnuts on a baking sheet and roast at 350°F (175°C) for 10-15 minutes, or until lightly toasted.

Usage:

Enjoy roasted walnuts as a snack to support brain health.

Benefits:

Walnuts provide alpha-linolenic acid and neuroprotective compounds, enhancing brain health and cognitive function.

393. Yerba Mate Energy Boost Tea

Description:

Yerba Mate provides a balanced energy boost along with nutrients that support mental functions.

Ingredients:

- 1 teaspoon yerba mate leaves or 1 yerba mate tea bag
- 1 cup boiling water
- Honey (optional, for sweetness)
- Lemon wedge (optional, for flavor)

Preparation Steps:

1. Steep yerba mate leaves or tea bag in boiling water for 5-10 minutes.
2. Strain the tea and let it cool to a safe drinking temperature.
3. Add honey and a lemon wedge if desired.

Usage:

Drink yerba mate tea in the morning or early afternoon for a balanced energy boost.

Benefits:

Yerba mate provides a natural energy boost and supports mental functions, promoting better focus and cognitive performance.

394. Custom Nootropic Stack Smoothie

Description:

A tailored blend of nootropics can be designed to meet individual needs for memory, focus, and cognitive speed.

Ingredients:

- 1 teaspoon custom nootropic blend (e.g., a mix of Bacopa Monnieri, Rhodiola Rosea, and Lion's Mane)
- 1 cup unsweetened almond milk
- 1 banana
- 1 tablespoon almond butter
- 1 tablespoon honey (optional, for sweetness)
- A handful of ice cubes

Preparation Steps:

Blend the custom nootropic blend, almond milk, banana, almond butter, honey, and ice cubes until smooth.

Usage:

Enjoy this nootropic stack smoothie in the morning to support memory, focus, and cognitive speed.

Benefits:

A custom blend of nootropics tailored to individual needs can enhance memory, focus, and cognitive speed, supporting overall brain health and mental clarity.

BONE AND JOINT HEALTH REMEDIES

395. Calcium-Rich Smoothie

Description:

This smoothie provides a bone-strengthening drink rich in calcium, supporting overall bone health.

Ingredients:

- 1 cup kale

- ☐ 1/2 cup plain yogurt
- ☐ 1 banana
- ☐ 1 tablespoon almond butter
- ☐ 1/2 cup almond milk

Preparation Steps:

1. Blend kale, yogurt, banana, almond butter, and almond milk until smooth.

Usage:

Enjoy this calcium-rich smoothie in the morning to support bone health.

Benefits:

This smoothie is rich in calcium and other essential nutrients, promoting strong bones and preventing osteoporosis.

396. Turmeric and Ginger Tea

Description:

This tea combines turmeric and ginger, known for their anti-inflammatory properties, to support joint health.

Ingredients:

- ☐ 1 teaspoon turmeric powder
- ☐ 1-inch fresh ginger root (sliced)
- ☐ 1 tablespoon honey
- ☐ Juice of 1 lemon

Preparation Steps:

1. Boil ginger in water for 10 minutes.
2. Add turmeric and simmer for an additional 10 minutes.
3. Strain the tea and add honey and lemon juice.

Usage:

Drink this turmeric and ginger tea daily to reduce inflammation and support joint health.

Benefits:

Turmeric and ginger help reduce inflammation and joint pain, promoting overall joint health and mobility.

397. Homemade Bone Broth

Description:

Bone broth is rich in collagen and minerals that support bone and joint health.

Ingredients:

- ☐ 2 pounds mixed beef bones
- ☐ 2 carrots (chopped)
- ☐ 1 onion (chopped)
- ☐ 2 celery stalks (chopped)
- ☐ 2 tablespoons apple cider vinegar

Preparation Steps:

1. Roast bones at 400°F for 30 minutes.
2. Simmer roasted bones with vegetables and vinegar in water for 24-48 hours.
3. Strain the broth and store.

Usage:

Drink bone broth daily or use it as a base for soups and stews to support bone and joint health.

Benefits:

Bone broth provides collagen and essential minerals that strengthen bones and support joint health.

398. Omega-3 Fish Oil Capsules

Description:

Fish oil capsules reduce inflammation and support joint lubrication.

Usage:

Take fish oil capsules daily as directed on the packaging to reduce inflammation and support joint health.

Benefits:

Omega-3 fatty acids in fish oil reduce inflammation and improve joint lubrication, promoting better joint mobility and reducing pain.

399. Magnesium Oil Spray for Joint Pain

Description:

Magnesium oil spray helps alleviate joint pain and support muscle function.

Ingredients:

- 1/2 cup magnesium chloride flakes
- 1/2 cup distilled water

Preparation Steps:

1. Heat water and dissolve magnesium flakes.
2. Cool the mixture and transfer to a spray bottle.

Usage:

Apply the magnesium oil spray topically to sore joints as needed.

Benefits:

Magnesium oil helps relieve joint pain and supports muscle function, promoting overall joint health.

400. Dried Plum Compote

Description:

Dried plums help improve bone density and support overall bone health.

Ingredients:

- 1 pound dried plums

- 1 cinnamon stick
- 2 cups water

Preparation Steps:

1. Simmer plums with cinnamon in water until soft.

Usage:

Eat dried plum compote daily to support bone health.

Benefits:

Dried plums are rich in nutrients that help improve bone density and support overall bone health.

401. Glucosamine & Chondroitin Supplement

Description:

This supplement supports cartilage health and joint mobility.

Usage:

Take the supplement daily as directed on the packaging to support joint health.

Benefits:

Glucosamine and chondroitin support cartilage health and improve joint mobility, reducing joint pain and stiffness.

402. Sesame Seed Sprinkle

Description:

Sesame seeds provide calcium and zinc, essential for bone health.

Preparation Steps:

Sprinkle toasted sesame seeds over salads or stir-fries.

Usage:

Incorporate sesame seeds into your meals to

support bone health.

Benefits:

Sesame seeds are rich in calcium and zinc, essential for maintaining strong bones and preventing osteoporosis.

403. Green Leafy Vegetable Stir-Fry

Description:

This stir-fry combines nutrient-rich greens to support bone health.

Ingredients:

- Spinach
- Kale
- Collard greens
- Garlic
- Olive oil

Preparation Steps:

1. Sauté garlic in olive oil.
2. Add spinach, kale, and collard greens, and cook until just wilted.

Usage:

Enjoy this stir-fry as a side dish to support bone health.

Benefits:

Green leafy vegetables provide essential vitamins and minerals that support bone health and overall well-being.

404. Herbal Joint Cream

Description:

This cream helps reduce pain and swelling in the joints.

Ingredients:

- Shea butter
- Beeswax
- Eucalyptus oil
- Ginger oil

Preparation Steps:

1. Melt shea butter with beeswax.
2. Stir in eucalyptus and ginger oils.
3. Cool and transfer to a jar.

Usage:

Apply the herbal joint cream to sore joints as needed.

Benefits:

This cream helps reduce joint pain and swelling, promoting better joint health and mobility.

405. Nettle Tea for Joint Health

Description:

Brew dried nettle leaves to create a mineral-rich tea that supports joint protection and reduces inflammation.

Ingredients:

- 1 teaspoon dried nettle leaves
- 1 cup boiling water
- Honey (optional, for sweetness)

Preparation Steps:

1. Steep dried nettle leaves in boiling water for 10-15 minutes.
2. Strain the tea and let it cool to a safe drinking temperature.
3. Add honey if desired.

Usage:

Drink a cup of nettle tea daily to support joint health and reduce inflammation.

Benefits:

Nettle tea is rich in minerals that support joint health and reduce inflammation, promoting overall joint protection.

406. Vitamin K2 MK-7 Supplement

Description:

Vitamin K2 MK-7 helps calcium deposit in the correct areas and enhances bone strength.

Usage:

Take the supplement daily as directed on the packaging to support bone health.

Benefits:

Vitamin K2 MK-7 ensures calcium is deposited in bones rather than arteries, enhancing bone strength and preventing cardiovascular issues.

407. Apple Cider Vinegar Tonic

Description:

This tonic helps support joint health and reduce inflammation.

Ingredients:

- 2 tablespoons apple cider vinegar
- 1 glass of water
- Honey to taste

Preparation Steps:

1. Mix apple cider vinegar with water.
2. Add honey to taste.

Usage:

Drink this apple cider vinegar tonic daily to support joint health.

Benefits:

Apple cider vinegar helps reduce inflammation and supports joint health, promoting overall well-being.

408. Boron Supplement

Description:

Boron helps increase bone density and reduce arthritis symptoms.

Usage:

Take the boron supplement daily as directed on the packaging to support bone health.

Benefits:

Boron increases bone density and reduces arthritis symptoms, promoting better joint and bone health.

409. Pineapple Bromelain Smoothie

Description:

This anti-inflammatory smoothie aids joint health and reduces inflammation.

Ingredients:

- 1 cup pineapple
- 1/2 cup Greek yogurt
- 1 teaspoon honey

Preparation Steps:

1. Blend pineapple, Greek yogurt, and honey until smooth.

Usage:

Enjoy this pineapple bromelain smoothie daily to support joint health.

Benefits:

Pineapple contains bromelain, an enzyme with anti-inflammatory properties that helps reduce joint pain and inflammation.

410. Rosehip Tea for Collagen Formation

Description:

Rosehip tea is rich in vitamin C, which helps collagen formation for joint and bone health.

Ingredients:

- 1 teaspoon dried rosehip
- 1 cup boiling water
- Honey (optional, for sweetness)

Preparation Steps:

1. Steep dried rosehip in boiling water for 10-15 minutes.
2. Strain the tea and let it cool to a safe drinking temperature.
3. Add honey if desired.

Usage:

Drink a cup of rosehip tea daily to support collagen formation and joint health.

Benefits:

Rosehip tea provides vitamin C, essential for collagen formation and joint health, promoting strong bones and joints.

411. Ginger Compress for Inflammation

Description:

A ginger compress helps reduce inflammation and soothe painful joints.

Ingredients:

- 1 tablespoon grated ginger
- Hot water
- Cloth

Preparation Steps:

1. Soak grated ginger in hot water for a few minutes.
2. Wrap the soaked ginger in a cloth.

Usage:

Apply the ginger compress to painful joints for 10-15 minutes to reduce inflammation.

Benefits:

Ginger has anti-inflammatory properties that help soothe and reduce pain in joints, promoting better joint health.

412. Flaxseed Oil Dressing for Joint Health

Description:

This salad dressing incorporates omega-3s that support joint health.

Ingredients:

- 1/4 cup flaxseed oil
- 2 tablespoons lemon juice
- 1 clove minced garlic
- 1 teaspoon mustard

Preparation Steps:

1. Whisk flaxseed oil, lemon juice, minced garlic, and mustard until well combined.

Usage:

Use this flaxseed oil dressing on salads to incorporate omega-3s into your diet.

Benefits:

Flaxseed oil provides omega-3 fatty acids that support joint health and reduce inflammation, promoting overall joint well-being.

413. Curcumin Supplements for Anti-Inflammatory Effects

Description:

Curcumin, combined with piperine, provides powerful anti-inflammatory effects that protect bones and joints.

Usage:

Take the supplement daily as directed on the packaging to benefit from anti-inflammatory effects.

Benefits:

Curcumin reduces inflammation and protects bones and joints, promoting better overall joint health.

414. Chili Pepper Capsaicin Cream for Pain Relief

Description:

Capsaicin cream relieves pain by depleting nerve endings of substance P.

Usage:

Apply the capsaicin cream topically to the skin over painful joints as directed on the packaging.

Benefits:

Capsaicin cream provides pain relief by depleting substance P from nerve endings, reducing joint pain and discomfort.

415. Moringa Leaf Powder Smoothie

Description:

Moringa leaf powder is rich in calcium and has anti-inflammatory properties, making it an excellent addition to smoothies for bone and joint health.

Ingredients:

- 1 teaspoon moringa leaf powder
- 1 banana
- 1 cup unsweetened almond milk
- 1/2 cup spinach
- 1 tablespoon honey (optional, for sweetness)
- A handful of ice cubes

Preparation Steps:

Blend moringa leaf powder, banana, almond milk, spinach, honey, and ice cubes until smooth.

Usage:

Enjoy this moringa smoothie in the morning or as a snack to support bone health and reduce inflammation.

Benefits:

Moringa powder provides calcium and anti-inflammatory compounds that support bone and joint health, promoting overall well-being.

416. Walnut and Dried Cherry Trail Mix

Description:

This trail mix is rich in antioxidants and anti-inflammatory compounds, supporting joint health and reducing inflammation.

Ingredients:

- 1 cup walnuts
- 1/2 cup dried cherries

□   1/2 cup dark chocolate chips

Preparation Steps:

1.   Mix walnuts, dried cherries, and dark chocolate chips in a bowl.

Usage:

Enjoy this trail mix as a healthy snack to support joint health and reduce inflammation.

Benefits:

Walnuts and dried cherries provide antioxidants and anti-inflammatory compounds that support joint health, while dark chocolate chips add a delicious touch.

417. Tart Cherry Juice for Inflammation

Description:

Tart cherry juice reduces joint inflammation and supports muscle recovery.

Usage:

Drink a glass of tart cherry juice daily to reduce inflammation and support muscle recovery.

Benefits:

Tart cherry juice is rich in anti-inflammatory compounds that help reduce joint pain and support muscle recovery, promoting overall joint health.

418. Epsom Salt Bath for Joint Pain

Description:

An Epsom salt bath helps relieve joint pain and stiffness through magnesium absorption.

Ingredients:

□   2 cups Epsom salts

□   Warm bathwater

Preparation Steps:

1.   Dissolve Epsom salts in warm bathwater.

Usage:

Soak in the Epsom salt bath for 20-30 minutes to relieve joint pain and stiffness.

Benefits:

Epsom salt baths provide magnesium, which helps relieve joint pain and reduce inflammation, promoting better joint health.

419. Collagen Peptide Powder for Joint Health

Description:

Collagen peptide powder supports joint and bone health through collagen synthesis.

Ingredients:

□   1 scoop collagen peptide powder

□   1 cup unsweetened almond milk (or preferred beverage)

□   1 banana (optional, for flavor)

□   1 tablespoon honey (optional, for sweetness)

□   A handful of ice cubes

Preparation Steps:

1.   Blend collagen peptide powder, almond milk, banana, honey, and ice cubes until smooth.

Usage:

Add collagen peptide powder to your morning smoothie or beverage to support joint and bone health.

Benefits:

Collagen peptides help support collagen synthesis, promoting stronger bones and healthier joints, reducing the risk of joint pain and stiffness.

RESPIRATORY HEALTH REMEDIES

420. Honey and Lemon Tea

Description:

Honey and lemon tea soothes the throat and reduces cough, making it a comforting remedy for respiratory health.

Ingredients:

- 1 tablespoon honey
- Juice of half a lemon
- 1 cup hot water

Preparation Steps:

1. Mix honey and lemon juice in hot water until well combined.

Usage:

Drink this honey and lemon tea to soothe the throat and reduce coughing.

Benefits:

Honey has antibacterial properties and soothes the throat, while lemon juice provides vitamin C and helps reduce inflammation, promoting respiratory health.

421. Peppermint Oil Steam Inhalation

Description:

Peppermint oil steam inhalation clears nasal passages and relieves congestion, supporting easier breathing.

Ingredients:

- 3-4 drops peppermint essential oil
- 1 pot boiling water

Preparation Steps:

1. Add peppermint oil to boiling water.
2. Inhale the steam by leaning over the pot with a towel draped over your head to trap the steam.

Usage:

Inhale the peppermint steam for 5-10 minutes to clear nasal passages and relieve congestion.

Benefits:

Peppermint oil helps clear nasal passages and reduce congestion, making it easier to breathe and supporting overall respiratory health.

422. Ginger Turmeric Tea

Description:

Ginger turmeric tea reduces inflammation and supports immune function, promoting respiratory health.

Ingredients:

- 1 inch fresh ginger (sliced)
- 1 teaspoon turmeric powder
- 1 tablespoon honey
- 1 liter water

Preparation Steps:

1. Boil ginger and turmeric in water.
2. Simmer for 10 minutes.
3. Strain the tea and add honey.

Usage:

Drink this ginger turmeric tea daily to reduce inflammation and support respiratory health.

Benefits:

Ginger and turmeric have anti-inflammatory properties, while honey soothes the throat, supporting immune function and reducing respiratory inflammation.

423. Eucalyptus Oil Chest Rub

Description:

Eucalyptus oil chest rub helps ease breathing and reduce cough by clearing airways.

Ingredients:

- 2 tablespoons coconut oil
- 5 drops eucalyptus essential oil

Preparation Steps:

1. Mix coconut oil and eucalyptus essential oil until well combined.

Usage:

Apply the eucalyptus oil chest rub to the chest and throat area to help ease breathing and reduce cough.

Benefits:

Eucalyptus oil helps clear airways and reduce cough, promoting easier breathing and respiratory comfort.

424. Licorice Root Tea

Description:

Licorice root tea soothes the throat and clears airways, supporting respiratory health.

Ingredients:

- 1 teaspoon dried licorice root
- 1 cup boiling water

Preparation Steps:

1. Steep licorice root in boiling water for 10 minutes.
2. Strain the tea.

Usage:

Drink this licorice root tea to soothe the throat and clear airways.

Benefits:

Licorice root helps soothe the throat and clear airways, promoting better respiratory health and comfort.

425. NAC (N-Acetyl Cysteine) Supplement

Description:

NAC helps thin mucus and improves the efficacy of the body's natural antioxidant defenses in the lungs.

Usage:

Take NAC supplements daily as directed on the packaging to support respiratory health.

Benefits:

NAC thins mucus and enhances antioxidant defenses in the lungs, promoting clearer airways and better respiratory health.

426. Mullein Leaf Tea

Description:

Mullein leaf tea supports healthy respiratory mucous membranes and clears the lungs.

Ingredients:

- 1 teaspoon dried mullein leaves
- 1 cup boiling water

Preparation Steps:

1. Steep mullein leaves in boiling water for 10 minutes.
2. Strain the tea.

Usage:

Drink this mullein leaf tea to support respiratory

health and clear the lungs.

Benefits:

Mullein leaf helps maintain healthy respiratory mucous membranes and clear the lungs, promoting better breathing and respiratory function.

427. Pine Needle Tea

Description:

Pine needle tea provides anti-inflammatory and antioxidant benefits, supporting respiratory health.

Ingredients:

- A handful of fresh pine needles
- 1 liter water

Preparation Steps:

1. Boil pine needles in water for 20 minutes.
2. Strain the tea.

Usage:

Drink this pine needle tea to benefit from its anti-inflammatory and antioxidant properties.

Benefits:

Pine needle tea supports respiratory health by reducing inflammation and providing antioxidants, promoting clearer airways and better breathing.

428. Thyme Infused Honey

Description:

Thyme infused honey relieves cough and soothes the throat, supporting respiratory comfort.

Ingredients:

- 1/2 cup honey
- 1 tablespoon dried thyme

Preparation Steps:

1. Gently warm honey and stir in dried thyme.
2. Let infuse for a week, then strain.

Usage:

Take a spoonful of thyme infused honey as needed to relieve cough and soothe the throat.

Benefits:

Thyme and honey provide antibacterial and soothing properties that help relieve cough and throat discomfort, promoting respiratory health.

429. Omega-3 Fatty Acids

Description:

Omega-3 fatty acids help reduce inflammation throughout the respiratory system.

Usage:

Take omega-3 fatty acid supplements daily as directed on the packaging to support respiratory health.

Benefits:

Omega-3 fatty acids reduce inflammation in the respiratory system, promoting clearer airways and better lung function.

430. Vitamin D Supplement

Description:

Daily vitamin D supplementation enhances immune function and reduces the risk of respiratory infections.

Usage:

Take the vitamin D supplement daily as directed on the packaging to support immune function.

Benefits:

Vitamin D helps enhance the immune system and reduce the risk of respiratory infections, promoting overall respiratory health.

431. Bromelain Supplement

Description:

Bromelain helps reduce mucus thickness and relieve sinusitis, supporting respiratory comfort.

Usage:

Take the bromelain supplement daily as directed on the packaging to help reduce mucus and relieve sinusitis.

Benefits:

Bromelain reduces mucus thickness and alleviates sinusitis, promoting clearer airways and better respiratory health.

432. Saline Nasal Spray

Description:

Saline nasal spray moisturizes nasal passages and helps clear out allergens and pathogens.

Usage:

Use the saline nasal spray regularly as directed on the packaging to keep nasal passages moist and clear.

Benefits:

Saline nasal spray helps maintain nasal hygiene by clearing out allergens and pathogens, supporting overall respiratory health.

433. Hot Peppers or Cayenne Pepper

Description:

Capsaicin in hot peppers acts as a natural decongestant, helping to clear nasal passages.

Ingredients:

Include small amounts of hot peppers or cayenne pepper in meals

Usage:

Incorporate hot peppers or cayenne pepper into your meals to leverage their natural decongestant properties.

Benefits:

Capsaicin in hot peppers helps clear nasal passages and reduce congestion, promoting easier breathing and respiratory comfort.

434. Chicken Soup for Respiratory Health

Description:

Chicken soup helps reduce respiratory symptoms and improve hydration, providing comfort during respiratory distress.

Ingredients:

- Chicken
- Carrots
- Celery
- Onions
- Garlic
- Herbs
- Water

Preparation Steps:

Simmer chicken, carrots, celery, onions, garlic, and herbs in water until the vegetables and chicken are cooked.

Usage:

Eat hot chicken soup to reduce respiratory symptoms and stay hydrated.

Benefits:

Chicken soup provides warmth, hydration, and

nutrients that help reduce respiratory symptoms and support overall health.

435. Slippery Elm Lozenges

Description:

Slippery elm lozenges soothe irritated throats and coughs, providing respiratory comfort.

Usage:

Use slippery elm lozenges as directed on the packaging to soothe the throat and reduce coughing.

Benefits:

Slippery elm lozenges provide soothing relief for irritated throats and coughs, promoting respiratory comfort and health.

436. Osha Root Tincture

Description:

Osha root tincture helps increase lung circulation and improve oxygenation during respiratory stress.

Usage:

Take the Osha root tincture as directed on the packaging to support lung circulation and oxygenation.

Benefits:

Osha root tincture enhances lung circulation and improves oxygenation, supporting better respiratory health during stress.

437. Astragalus Root Supplement

Description:

Astragalus root strengthens the immune system and supports lung health, promoting overall respiratory well-being.

Usage:

Take the Astragalus root supplement regularly as directed on the packaging to support the immune system and lung health.

Benefits:

Astragalus root helps strengthen the immune system and support lung health, promoting overall respiratory wellness.

438. Air-Purifying Plants

Description:

Keeping air-purifying plants like snake plant, spider plant, or peace lily indoors helps remove toxins from the air.

Ingredients:

- Snake plant, spider plant, or peace lily

Usage:

Place air-purifying plants in indoor spaces to improve air quality.

Benefits:

Air-purifying plants help remove toxins from the air, improving indoor air quality and supporting better respiratory health.

439. Andrographis Supplement

Description:

Andrographis is known for its immune-boosting and anti-inflammatory properties, helpful in preventing and easing respiratory infections.

Usage:

Take the Andrographis supplement as directed on the packaging to boost the immune system and reduce inflammation.

Benefits:

Andrographis helps prevent respiratory infections and ease symptoms, promoting overall respiratory health.

440. Essential Oil Diffuser with a Blend of Rosemary and Lemon

Description:

Using an essential oil diffuser with a blend of rosemary and lemon helps purify the air and provide respiratory relief.

Ingredients:

- 3-4 drops rosemary essential oil
- 3-4 drops lemon essential oil
- Essential oil diffuser

Preparation Steps:

1. Add rosemary and lemon essential oils to the diffuser.
2. Fill the diffuser with water according to the manufacturer's instructions.

Usage:

Use the diffuser in your living environment to purify the air and support respiratory health.

Benefits:

The blend of rosemary and lemon essential oils helps purify the air, relieve respiratory discomfort, and promote easier breathing.

441. Lobelia Extract for Breathing Ease

Description:

Lobelia extract, used cautiously, acts as a bronchodilator to help ease breathing in acute respiratory distress.

Usage:

Take lobelia extract as directed on the packaging, preferably under medical supervision, to ease breathing during respiratory distress.

Benefits:

Lobelia extract helps dilate the bronchi, improving airflow and easing breathing during acute respiratory distress.

442. Cordyceps Mushroom Supplements

Description:

Cordyceps mushrooms increase oxygen uptake and boost cellular immunity, beneficial for lung health.

Usage:

Take cordyceps supplements daily as directed on the packaging to support lung health.

Benefits:

Cordyceps mushrooms enhance oxygen uptake and boost immunity, supporting better lung function and overall respiratory health.

443. Elecampane Root Tea for Lung Detoxification

Description:

Elecampane root tea supports lung detoxification and mucus clearance.

Ingredients:

- 1 teaspoon dried elecampane root
- 1 cup water

Preparation Steps:

1. Boil dried elecampane root in water for 10 minutes.
2. Strain the tea.

Usage:

Drink elecampane root tea daily to support lung health and clear mucus.

Benefits:

Elecampane root helps detoxify the lungs and clear mucus, promoting better respiratory function and lung health.

444. Quercetin Supplement for Respiratory Health

Description:

Quercetin helps stabilize mast cells and reduce the frequency of respiratory flare-ups due to its antioxidant properties.

Usage:

Take quercetin supplements daily as directed on the packaging to support respiratory health.

Benefits:

Quercetin's antioxidant properties help stabilize mast cells and reduce respiratory flare-ups, promoting overall respiratory well-being.

EYE HEALTH REMEDIES

445. Carrot and Ginger Juice for Vision

Description:

Carrot and ginger juice is rich in beta-carotene and antioxidants, vital for good vision and eye health.

Ingredients:

- 2 large carrots
- 1-inch piece of ginger
- 1 apple

Preparation Steps:

1. Juice the carrots, ginger, and apple together.

Usage:

Drink this carrot and ginger juice daily to support eye health and improve vision.

Benefits:

Beta-carotene from carrots and antioxidants from ginger and apple support good vision and overall eye health.

446. Bilberry Extract for Night Vision

Description:

Bilberry extract improves night vision and overall eye health due to its high levels of anthocyanins.

Usage:

Take bilberry supplements daily as directed on the packaging to support eye health.

Benefits:

Bilberry extract contains anthocyanins that improve night vision and overall eye health, promoting better vision clarity.

447. Omega-3 Fatty Acids for Retinal Health

Description:

Omega-3 fatty acids support retinal health and prevent dry eye syndrome.

Usage:

Take omega-3 supplements daily as directed on

the packaging to support retinal health.

Benefits:

Omega-3 fatty acids maintain retinal health and prevent dry eye syndrome, promoting better overall eye function.

448. Green Leafy Vegetable Salad for Eye Health

Description:

This salad is high in lutein and zeaxanthin, important nutrients for eye health.

Ingredients:

- Spinach
- Kale
- Swiss chard
- Olive oil
- Lemon juice

Preparation Steps:

1. Toss fresh spinach, kale, and Swiss chard in olive oil and lemon juice.

Usage:

Enjoy this salad regularly to support eye health.

Benefits:

Lutein and zeaxanthin in green leafy vegetables help protect the eyes from damage and improve overall eye health.

449. Zinc-Rich Trail Mix for Retina Support

Description:

This trail mix is rich in zinc, supporting the retina and reducing the risk of macular degeneration.

Ingredients:

- Pumpkin seeds
- Cashews
- Dark chocolate chips

Preparation Steps:

1. Mix pumpkin seeds, cashews, and dark chocolate chips together.

Usage:

Enjoy this zinc-rich trail mix as a healthy snack to support eye health.

Benefits:

Zinc supports retinal health and helps reduce the risk of macular degeneration, promoting better eye function.

450. Vitamin A Fortified Smoothie

Description:

This smoothie is rich in vitamin A, essential for maintaining healthy corneas.

Ingredients:

- 1/2 cup mango
- 1/2 cup cantaloupe
- 1 cup fortified almond milk

Preparation Steps:

1. Blend mango, cantaloupe, and fortified almond milk until smooth.

Usage:

Drink this vitamin A fortified smoothie regularly to support eye health.

Benefits:

Vitamin A helps maintain healthy corneas and improves overall eye health, promoting better vision.

Beta-carotene in sweet potatoes promotes good vision and overall eye health, reducing the risk of eye diseases.

451. Selenium-Rich Brazil Nuts for Cataract Prevention

Description:

Brazil nuts provide selenium, an antioxidant that plays a key role in preventing cataracts.

Ingredients:

- 1-2 Brazil nuts

Usage:

1. Eat 1-2 Brazil nuts daily to get selenium.

Benefits:

Selenium helps prevent cataracts and supports overall eye health, promoting better vision clarity.

452. Sweet Potato Fries for Vision

Description:

Sweet potatoes are high in beta-carotene, promoting good vision and eye health.

Ingredients:

- Sweet potatoes
- Olive oil
- Salt

Preparation Steps:

1. Slice sweet potatoes, toss in olive oil and salt, and bake until crispy.

Usage:

Enjoy sweet potato fries as a healthy snack to support vision.

Benefits:

453. Goji Berry Snack for Macular Protection

Description:

Goji berries are known for their high levels of zeaxanthin, which protects against macular degeneration.

Ingredients:

A small handful of goji berries

Usage:

Eat a small handful of goji berries daily.

Benefits:

Zeaxanthin in goji berries protects against macular degeneration and supports overall eye health.

454. Egg Spinach Omelette for Eye Health

Description:

Eggs and spinach are great sources of lutein and zeaxanthin, beneficial for eye health.

Ingredients:

- Eggs
- Spinach
- Olive oil

Preparation Steps:

1. Cook spinach in olive oil until wilted.
2. Add beaten eggs and cook until set.

Usage:

Enjoy this egg spinach omelette regularly to support eye health.

Benefits:

Lutein and zeaxanthin in eggs and spinach help protect the eyes from damage and improve overall eye health.

455. Vitamin C Citrus Salad

Description:

Vitamin C helps form and maintain collagen found in the cornea, promoting eye health.

Ingredients:

- Oranges
- Grapefruits
- Lemon zest

Preparation Steps:

Combine citrus fruits in a bowl and sprinkle with lemon zest.

Usage:

Enjoy this citrus salad regularly to support collagen formation and overall eye health.

Benefits:

This salad is rich in vitamin C, essential for maintaining collagen in the cornea and promoting healthy vision.

456. Broccoli and Pepper Stir-Fry

Description:

Broccoli and bell peppers are rich in vitamin C, which supports eye health.

Ingredients:

- Broccoli
- Bell peppers
- Garlic
- Soy sauce

Preparation Steps:

1. Stir-fry broccoli, bell peppers, and garlic in soy sauce.

Usage:

Enjoy this stir-fry as a nutritious meal to support eye health.

Benefits:

The high vitamin C content in broccoli and bell peppers helps protect the eyes and maintain healthy vision.

457. Chia Seed Pudding

Description:

Chia seeds are high in omega-3, which is good for eye moisture.

Ingredients:

- Chia seeds
- Almond milk
- Honey

Preparation Steps:

1. Mix chia seeds with almond milk and honey.
2. Let sit until thickened.

Usage:

Enjoy this chia seed pudding as a healthy snack or breakfast to support eye moisture.

Benefits:

Omega-3 fatty acids in chia seeds help maintain eye moisture and reduce the risk of dry eye syndrome.

458. Saffron Risotto

Description:

Saffron may protect against eye diseases and improve vision.

Ingredients:

- Arborio rice
- Chicken broth
- Saffron
- Parmesan cheese

Preparation Steps:

1. Cook rice in chicken broth, adding saffron.
2. Finish with parmesan cheese.

Usage:

Enjoy this saffron risotto as a flavorful dish to support eye health.

Benefits:

Saffron contains compounds that may protect against eye diseases and improve overall vision.

459 Rosemary Roasted Almonds

Description:

Almonds contain vitamin E, which slows macular degeneration.

Ingredients:

- Almonds
- Rosemary
- Olive oil

Preparation Steps:

1. Roast almonds with rosemary and olive oil.

Usage:

Enjoy these rosemary roasted almonds as a healthy snack to support eye health.

Benefits:

Vitamin E in almonds helps slow macular degeneration and supports overall eye health.

460. Tuna Salad

Description:

Tuna is rich in omega-3 fatty acids, crucial for eye health.

Ingredients:

- Canned tuna
- Mayonnaise
- Celery
- Onion

Preparation Steps:

1. Mix tuna, mayonnaise, celery, and onion together.

Usage:

Enjoy this tuna salad regularly to support eye health.

Benefits:

Omega-3 fatty acids in tuna help maintain retinal health and prevent dry eye syndrome.

461. Kale Chips

Description:

Kale is a great source of lutein and zeaxanthin, important for eye health.

Ingredients:

- Kale leaves
- Olive oil
- Salt

Preparation Steps:

1. Toss kale in olive oil and salt.

2. Bake until crisp.

Usage:

Enjoy these kale chips as a nutritious snack to support eye health.

Benefits:

Lutein and zeaxanthin in kale help protect the eyes from damage and improve overall vision health.

462. Watercress Soup

Description:

Watercress is high in vitamin C and antioxidants, supporting eye health.

Ingredients:

- Watercress
- Potatoes
- Vegetable broth
- Onions

Preparation Steps:

1. Simmer watercress, potatoes, vegetable broth, and onions until tender.
2. Blend until smooth.

Usage:

Enjoy this watercress soup as a nutritious meal to support eye health.

Benefits:

Vitamin C and antioxidants in watercress help protect the eyes and maintain healthy vision.

463. Papaya Smoothie

Description:

Papaya is high in vitamin C and beta-carotene, promoting good vision.

Ingredients:

- Papaya
- Coconut water
- Lime juice

Preparation Steps:

1. Blend papaya, coconut water, and lime juice until smooth.

Usage:

Enjoy this papaya smoothie regularly to support eye health.

Benefits:

Vitamin C and beta-carotene in papaya help maintain healthy vision and protect the eyes from damage.

464. Blueberry Yogurt Parfait

Description:

Blueberries are known for their role in improving night vision.

Ingredients:

- Blueberries
- Plain yogurt
- Honey

Preparation Steps:

1. Layer blueberries and yogurt in a glass.
2. Drizzle with honey.

Usage:

Enjoy this blueberry yogurt parfait as a nutritious snack or breakfast to support eye health.

Benefits:

Blueberries contain antioxidants that improve night vision and support overall eye health.

465. Tomato Basil Soup

Description:

Tomatoes are rich in vitamin C and lycopene, important for eye health.

Ingredients:

- Tomatoes
- Basil
- Vegetable broth
- Cream

Preparation Steps:

1. Cook tomatoes and basil in vegetable broth.
2. Blend until smooth.
3. Add cream and stir until well combined.

Usage:

Enjoy this tomato basil soup regularly to support eye health.

Benefits:

Vitamin C and lycopene in tomatoes help protect the eyes and support overall vision health.

466. Roasted Bell Peppers

Description:

Bell peppers are high in vitamin C, which supports eye health.

Ingredients:

- Bell peppers
- Olive oil
- Garlic

Preparation Steps:

1. Slice bell peppers and toss with olive oil and garlic.

2. Roast until tender.

Usage:

Enjoy roasted bell peppers as a nutritious side dish to support eye health.

Benefits:

Vitamin C in bell peppers helps protect the eyes and maintain healthy vision.

467. Cod Liver Oil Supplement

Description:

Cod liver oil is a direct source of vitamins A and D, crucial for eye health.

Usage:

Take cod liver oil capsules daily as directed on the packaging to support eye health.

Benefits:

Vitamins A and D in cod liver oil help maintain healthy vision and support overall eye health.

468. Lutein and Zeaxanthin Supplement

Description:

Lutein and zeaxanthin are crucial carotenoids for eye health.

Usage:

Take lutein and zeaxanthin supplements daily as directed on the packaging to ensure adequate intake.

Benefits:

These carotenoids protect the eyes from damage and support healthy vision, reducing the risk of eye diseases.

468. Sunflower Seeds Snack

Description:

Sunflower seeds are rich in vitamin E and selenium, which support good eye health.

Usage:

Eat sunflower seeds as a snack to support eye health.

Benefits:

Vitamin E and selenium in sunflower seeds help protect the eyes and maintain overall eye health.

ALLERGY RELIEF REMEDIES

469. Local Honey for Allergy Relief

Description:

Local honey contains local pollen, which can help desensitize your body to allergens.

Consumption:

Take 1 tablespoon of local honey daily.

Usage:

Consume local honey daily to help your body build immunity against local allergens.

Benefits:

Local honey helps desensitize your body to pollen, reducing allergy symptoms and providing natural relief.

470. Nettle Tea for Allergy Relief

Description:

Nettle tea reduces histamine production, helping to alleviate allergy symptoms.

Ingredients:

Dried nettle leaves

Preparation Steps:

Steep dried nettle leaves in hot water for 10 minutes.

Usage:

Drink nettle tea daily during allergy season to reduce histamine production.

Benefits:

Nettle tea acts as a natural antihistamine, reducing allergy symptoms and promoting relief.

471. Quercetin Supplement for Allergy Relief

Description:

Quercetin is a natural antihistamine and anti-inflammatory that can reduce symptoms of seasonal allergies.

Consumption:

Take quercetin supplements as directed on the packaging.

Usage:

Take quercetin supplements daily to alleviate allergy symptoms.

Benefits:

Quercetin helps reduce inflammation and histamine production, providing relief from seasonal allergies.

472. Bromelain Smoothie for Allergy Relief

Description:

Bromelain in pineapple can help reduce nasal

swelling and other symptoms of allergies.

Ingredients:

- Pineapple chunks (rich in bromelain)
- Coconut water
- Spinach

Preparation Steps:

Blend pineapple chunks, coconut water, and spinach until smooth.

Usage:

Drink this bromelain smoothie to reduce nasal swelling and alleviate allergy symptoms.

Benefits:

Bromelain reduces inflammation and nasal swelling, promoting better respiratory health and relief from allergy symptoms.

473. Peppermint Tea for Congestion Relief

Description:

Peppermint tea relieves nasal and respiratory congestion, helping to alleviate allergy symptoms.

Ingredients:

Peppermint leaves

Preparation Steps:

1. Steep peppermint leaves in hot water for 10 minutes.

Usage:

Drink peppermint tea to relieve nasal and respiratory congestion.

Benefits:

Peppermint tea helps clear nasal passages and reduce congestion, providing relief from allergy symptoms.

474. Eucalyptus Oil Steam Inhalation

Description:

Eucalyptus oil steam inhalation clears nasal passages and relieves congestion.

Ingredients:

- Eucalyptus essential oil
- Hot water

Preparation Steps:

1. Add a few drops of eucalyptus oil to a bowl of hot water.
2. Inhale the steam by leaning over the bowl with a towel draped over your head to trap the steam.

Usage:

Inhale eucalyptus steam for 5-10 minutes to clear nasal passages.

Benefits:

Eucalyptus steam helps reduce nasal congestion and clear airways, providing relief from allergy symptoms.

475. Omega-3 Fatty Acids for Allergy Relief

Description:

Omega-3 fatty acids help reduce inflammation associated with allergic reactions.

Consumption:

Take fish oil or flaxseed oil supplements daily as directed on the packaging.

Usage:

Consume omega-3 fatty acids regularly to reduce inflammation and alleviate allergy symptoms.

Benefits:

Omega-3 fatty acids reduce inflammation, helping to alleviate symptoms of allergic reactions and support overall health.

476. Apple Cider Vinegar Drink for Immune Support

Description:

Apple cider vinegar boosts the immune system and alleviates allergy symptoms.

Ingredients:

- 2 teaspoons apple cider vinegar
- 1 glass water
- Honey to taste

Preparation Steps:

1. Mix apple cider vinegar and honey in water.

Usage:

Drink this apple cider vinegar mixture daily to support the immune system and alleviate allergy symptoms.

Benefits:

Apple cider vinegar helps boost the immune system and reduce allergy symptoms, promoting better overall health.

477. Spirulina Smoothie for Allergy Relief

Description:

Spirulina may reduce the release of histamine from mast cells, alleviating allergy symptoms.

Ingredients:

- 1 teaspoon spirulina powder
- 1 banana
- 1 cup almond milk

Preparation Steps:

1. Blend spirulina powder, banana, and almond milk until smooth.

Usage:

Drink this spirulina smoothie to reduce histamine release and alleviate allergy symptoms.

Benefits:

Spirulina helps reduce histamine release, promoting relief from allergy symptoms and supporting overall health.

478. Turmeric Milk for Inflammation Relief

Description:

Turmeric milk utilizes turmeric's anti-inflammatory properties to alleviate allergy symptoms.

Ingredients:

- 1 teaspoon turmeric powder
- 1 cup milk or a milk alternative
- Honey to taste

Preparation Steps:

1. Heat the milk and stir in turmeric and honey.

Usage:

Drink this turmeric milk to reduce inflammation and alleviate allergy symptoms.

Benefits:

Turmeric's anti-inflammatory properties help reduce allergy symptoms and promote overall respiratory health.

479. Butterbur Supplement for Allergy Relief

Description:

Butterbur helps relieve nasal symptoms of hay fever without causing drowsiness.

Consumption:

Take butterbur supplements as directed on the packaging.

Usage:

Consume butterbur supplements daily during allergy season to reduce nasal symptoms.

Benefits:

Butterbur provides relief from hay fever symptoms without the side effects of drowsiness, promoting better respiratory health.

480. Ginger Lemon Honey Tea for Throat Irritation

Description:

Ginger lemon honey tea alleviates throat irritation and provides soothing relief.

Ingredients:

- 1 inch ginger root
- Juice of 1 lemon
- 1 tablespoon honey
- 1 cup water

Preparation Steps:

1. Boil ginger in water.
2. Add lemon juice and honey.
3. Stir well.

Usage:

Drink this ginger lemon honey tea to soothe throat irritation.

Benefits:

Ginger, lemon, and honey work together to soothe the throat and reduce irritation, providing relief from allergy symptoms.

481. Probiotics for Gut Health and Immune Function

Description:

Probiotics support gut health and enhance immune function, helping to alleviate allergy symptoms.

Consumption:

Take probiotics through supplements or fermented foods like yogurt, kefir, and sauerkraut.

Usage:

Consume probiotics daily to support gut health and boost the immune system.

Benefits:

Probiotics help maintain a healthy gut microbiome and enhance immune function, reducing the severity of allergy symptoms.

482. Hot and Spicy Foods for Nasal Congestion

Description:

Hot and spicy foods like cayenne pepper, garlic, and horseradish help thin mucus and clear nasal passages.

Consumption:

Incorporate hot and spicy foods into your meals regularly.

Usage:

Eat hot and spicy foods to relieve nasal congestion and improve breathing.

Benefits:

The capsaicin and other compounds in spicy foods thin mucus and clear nasal passages, providing relief from congestion.

483. Vitamin C Rich Foods for Immune Boost

Description:

Foods high in vitamin C help boost the immune system and act as natural antihistamines.

Consumption:

Eat foods rich in vitamin C like oranges, strawberries, and bell peppers.

Usage:

Consume vitamin C-rich foods daily to support immune function and reduce allergy symptoms.

Benefits:

Vitamin C boosts the immune system and acts as a natural antihistamine, providing relief from allergy symptoms.

484. Stinging Nettle Capsules for Hay Fever

Description:

Stinging nettle is a natural antihistamine that helps control hay fever symptoms.

Consumption:

Take stinging nettle capsules as directed on the packaging.

Usage:

Consume stinging nettle capsules during allergy season to reduce hay fever symptoms.

Benefits:

Stinging nettle reduces histamine production, alleviating hay fever symptoms and promoting respiratory comfort.

485. Nasal Saline Irrigation for Congestion Relief

Description:

Nasal saline irrigation helps flush out sinuses and relieve nasal congestion.

Preparation Steps:

1. Use a neti pot with a saline solution.
2. Tilt your head to one side and pour the saline solution into one nostril, allowing it to flow out of the other nostril.
3. Repeat on the other side.

Usage:

Perform nasal saline irrigation daily to clear sinuses and reduce congestion.

Benefits:

Saline irrigation helps remove allergens and mucus from the nasal passages, providing relief from congestion and improving breathing.

486. Chamomile Tea for Inflammation Relief

Description:

Chamomile tea acts as an anti-inflammatory, providing soothing relief from allergy symptoms.

Ingredients:

▫ Chamomile flowers

Preparation Steps:

1. Steep chamomile flowers in hot water for 10 minutes.

Usage:

Drink chamomile tea to reduce inflammation and soothe allergy symptoms.

Benefits:

Chamomile has anti-inflammatory properties that help reduce allergic inflammation and provide relief from symptoms.

487. Licorice Root Tea for Sore Throat Relief

Description:

Licorice root tea soothes sore throats and reduces allergic inflammation.

Ingredients:

▫ Dried licorice root

Preparation Steps:

1. Boil dried licorice root in water for 10 minutes.
2. Strain the tea.

Usage:

Drink licorice root tea to soothe sore throats and reduce inflammation.

Benefits:

Licorice root helps reduce throat irritation and allergic inflammation, providing relief from allergy symptoms.

488. Bee Pollen for Immunity to Local Pollens

Description:

Bee pollen can help build up immunity to local pollens, reducing allergy symptoms.

Consumption:

Start with small amounts of bee pollen and gradually increase the dose.

Usage:

Consume bee pollen daily to build immunity against local allergens.

Benefits:

Bee pollen helps desensitize the body to local pollens, reducing the severity of allergy symptoms and promoting better respiratory health.

489. Lavender Essential Oil for Allergy Relief and Sleep

Description:

Lavender essential oil helps reduce allergic reactions and promotes a soothing sleep environment.

Use:

Diffuse lavender oil in your bedroom at night.

Usage:

Add a few drops of lavender essential oil to a diffuser before bedtime.

Benefits:

Lavender oil helps reduce allergic reactions and promotes relaxation, supporting better sleep and overall well-being.

490. Mint Essential Oil for Congestion and Headache Relief

Description:

Mint essential oil helps clear congestion and relieve headaches, providing comfort during allergy season.

Use:

Add to a diffuser or place a few drops on a tissue for inhaling.

Usage:

Diffuse mint oil or inhale from a tissue to relieve nasal congestion and headaches.

Benefits:

Mint essential oil provides relief from nasal congestion and headaches, promoting clearer breathing and comfort.

491. HEPA Filter for Allergen Reduction

Description:

A HEPA filter helps filter out pollen, dust, and other allergens from the air, improving indoor air quality.

Use:

Install a HEPA filter in your home.

Usage:

Use the HEPA filter continuously to maintain clean air and reduce exposure to allergens.

Benefits:

A HEPA filter removes airborne allergens, promoting better respiratory health and reducing allergy symptoms.

492. Magnesium-Rich Foods for Immune Support

Description:

Magnesium-rich foods support immune system function and help reduce allergy symptoms.

Consumption:

Include almonds, spinach, and pumpkin seeds in your diet.

Usage:

Consume magnesium-rich foods regularly to support immune health.

Benefits:

Magnesium supports immune function and helps reduce inflammation, alleviating allergy symptoms and promoting overall health.

493. Goldenseal Supplement for Allergy Relief

Description:

Goldenseal has antibacterial and immune-boosting properties that help reduce allergy symptoms.

Consumption:

Take goldenseal supplements as directed on the packaging.

Usage:

Consume goldenseal supplements daily to support immune health and reduce allergy symptoms.

Benefits:

Goldenseal helps boost the immune system and provides antibacterial benefits, reducing the severity of allergy symptoms.

494. Turmeric Ginger Smoothie

Description:

This smoothie combines turmeric and ginger, both known for their anti-inflammatory properties, to help reduce allergy symptoms naturally.

Ingredients:

- 1 teaspoon turmeric powder
- 1 inch ginger root
- 1 banana
- 1 cup coconut milk
- Honey to taste

Preparation Steps:

1. Blend all ingredients until smooth.
2. Adjust honey for sweetness if needed.

Usage:

Drink this smoothie daily, especially during allergy season, to reduce inflammation and alleviate allergy symptoms.

Benefits:

Turmeric and ginger both have anti-inflammatory properties that can help reduce nasal swelling and other allergy symptoms, promoting overall respiratory health.

495. Elderberry Syrup

Description:

Elderberry syrup is a potent natural remedy for boosting the immune system and reducing inflammation, which can help manage allergy symptoms.

Ingredients:

- 1 cup dried elderberries
- 4 cups water
- 1 cup honey

Preparation Steps:

1. Simmer elderberries in water until the liquid is reduced by half.
2. Strain the mixture and mix the liquid with honey.

Usage:

Take 1 tablespoon of elderberry syrup daily to help boost immunity and reduce allergy-related inflammation.

Benefits:

Elderberries are rich in antioxidants and vitamins that strengthen the immune system and reduce inflammation, helping to alleviate symptoms of allergies.

496. Garlic Tea

Description:

Garlic tea leverages the natural antihistamine properties of garlic to help reduce allergy symptoms and improve respiratory health.

Ingredients:

- 2 cloves garlic, crushed
- 1 cup water
- Honey to taste

Preparation Steps:

1. Boil water and add crushed garlic.
2. Let steep for 10 minutes, then strain and add honey.

Usage:

Drink garlic tea daily during allergy season to help reduce symptoms and support respiratory health.

Benefits:

Garlic contains natural antihistamines that can help reduce allergy symptoms and improve overall respiratory function.

497. Carrot Juice

Description:

Carrot juice, rich in beta-carotene and antioxidants, can help reduce inflammation and improve immune function, making it effective for managing allergies.

Ingredients:

- 4 carrots
- 1 apple
- 1 inch ginger root

Preparation Steps:

1. Juice all ingredients together.
2. Mix well and serve fresh.

Usage:

Drink carrot juice daily to help reduce inflammation and support immune health during allergy season.

Benefits:

Carrots are high in beta-carotene, which reduces inflammation and improves immune response, helping to manage allergy symptoms.

498. Basil Tea

Description:

Basil tea offers anti-inflammatory benefits that can help alleviate allergy symptoms and promote respiratory health.

Ingredients:

- Fresh basil leaves
- 1 cup boiling water

Preparation Steps:

1. Steep fresh basil leaves in boiling water for 10 minutes.
2. Strain and serve hot.

Usage:

Drink basil tea daily to reduce inflammation and alleviate allergy symptoms.

Benefits:

Basil's anti-inflammatory properties help reduce nasal swelling and improve respiratory health, making it effective for managing allergies.

499. Mullein Tea

Description:

Mullein tea helps soothe respiratory issues and reduce mucus, providing relief from allergy symptoms.

Ingredients:

- 1 teaspoon dried mullein leaves
- 1 cup boiling water

Preparation Steps:

1. Steep dried mullein leaves in boiling water for 10 minutes.
2. Strain and serve hot.

Usage:

Drink mullein tea daily, especially during allergy season, to help clear mucus and soothe respiratory passages.

Benefits:

Mullein's soothing properties help reduce mucus and alleviate respiratory symptoms associated with allergies.

500. Rosemary Steam Inhalation

Description:

Rosemary steam inhalation helps open nasal passages and reduce congestion, providing relief from allergy symptoms.

Ingredients:

- Fresh rosemary sprigs
- 1 bowl boiling water

Preparation Steps:

1. Add rosemary to boiling water.
2. Inhale the steam for several minutes.

Usage:

Use rosemary steam inhalation daily to help clear nasal passages and reduce congestion.

Benefits:

Rosemary's natural decongestant properties help open nasal passages and improve breathing, reducing allergy symptoms.

CONCLUSION

As we draw this enlightening journey to a close, it is essential to reflect on the profound insights and practical wisdom that "The Outlive Natural Remedies Encyclopedia" has offered. This book is more than a collection of herbal recipes and health tips; it is a testament to the harmonious marriage of traditional natural remedies and modern scientific understanding, inspired by the meticulous teachings of Dr. Peter Attia.

Throughout these pages, we have explored the intricate dance between nature's pharmacy and the cutting-edge principles of longevity science. We've delved into how embracing natural remedies can foster an environment within our bodies that supports optimal health and delays the onset of age-related decline. This is not just about adding years to our lives but about adding life to our years—ensuring that each moment is lived with vitality, purpose, and well-being.

The knowledge shared here is designed to empower you to take control of your health journey. By integrating the natural remedies and lifestyle adjustments outlined in this book, you can align your daily practices with the principles of health optimization and preventive medicine. This approach is not about seeking quick fixes but about making sustained, meaningful changes that enhance your quality of life.

Remember, the journey to longevity and robust health is deeply personal and continuous. It requires a commitment to understanding and respecting the body's natural processes and supporting them with the best that nature and science have to offer. Whether you are new to these concepts or have been following them for years, let this book serve as your companion, guiding you towards a life characterized by health, balance, and resilience.

As you move forward, carry with you the insights and tools you have gained. Embrace the natural remedies that resonate with you, experiment with the recipes that nourish you, and adopt the lifestyle practices that enhance your well-being. Each small step you take is a stride towards a longer, healthier, and more fulfilling life.

In closing, let us celebrate the remarkable potential within each of us to thrive. With a heart open to nature's wisdom and a mind informed by scientific rigor, we can unlock the secrets to a life well-lived. May your journey be filled with discovery, growth, and the vibrant health that comes from living in harmony with the natural world and the innovative insights of longevity science.

Thank you for embarking on this journey with us. Here's to your health, longevity, and a life of endless possibilities.

Made in the USA
Las Vegas, NV
13 July 2024